Research on early developmental care for preterm neonates

ISBN 2-7420-0416-5

Éditions John Libbey Eurotext
127, avenue de la République
92120 Montrouge, France.
Tél. : 33 (0)1 46 73 06 60
e-mail: contact@jle.com
http://www.jle.com

John Libbey & Company Ltd
42-46 High Street
Esher Surrey
KT10 9QY
United Kingdom

Editor: Maud Thévenin

© John Libbey Eurotext, Paris, 2005

It is prohibited to reproduce this work or any part of it without authorisation of the publisher or of the Centre Français d'Exploitation du Droit de Copie (CFC), 20, rue des Grands-Augustins, 75006 Paris.

Research on early developmental care for preterm neonates

Jacques Sizun
Joy Browne

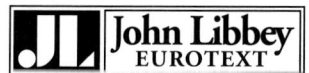

List of Contributors

Amiel-Tison Claudine, Port-Royal-Baudelocque, Paris, France
Bauer Karl, Department of Pediatrics, Klinikum der Johann Wolfgang-Goethe Universität, Frankfurt am Main, Germany
Browne Joy, University of Colorado, Department of Pediatrics, Denver, USA
Cazillis Michèle, INSERM E 9935, Hôpital Robert Debré, Paris, France
Coureaud Gérard, Centre des Sciences du Goût, UMR 5170 CNRS-Université de Bourgogne, Dijon, France
Cuttini Marina, Unità di Epidemiologia, Ospedale Pediatrico Bambino Gesù, Piazza S.Onofrio 4, Roma, Italy
Debillon Thierry, Service de Réanimation Pédiatrique, CHRU de Grenoble, France
Gosselin Julie, Université de Montréal, Canada
Goubet Nathalie, Department of Psychology, Gettysburg College, USA
Greisen Gorm, Department of Neonatalogy 5024, Rigshospitalet, Copenhague, Denmark
Gressens Pierre, INSERM E 9935 and Service de Neuropédiatrie, Hôpital Robert Debré, Paris, France
Hansen Valérie, Department of Neonatology, Neonatal Intensive Care Unit, St Pierre University Hospital, Rue Haute, 322, B-1000 Brussels, Belgium
Haumont Dominique, Department of Neonatology, Neonatal Intensive Care Unit, St Pierre University Hospital, Rue Haute, 322, B-1000 Brussels, Belgium
Hedberg Nyqvist Kerstin, RN PhD IBCLC, Assistant Professor in Pediatric Nursing, Department of Women's and Children's Health, Section for Pediatrics, Uppsala University, Uppsala, Sweden
Hellström-Westas Lena, Department of Pediatrics and Clinical Neurophysiology, Lund University Hospital, Sweden
Kleberg Agneta, Dept. of Woman and Child Health, Neonatal Programme, Karolinska Institute, Astrid Lindgren Children's Hospital, and Danderyd Hospital, Stockholm, Sweden and Dept. of Paediatrics, University of Lund, Lund, Sweden
Lagercrantz Hugo, Karolinska Institute, Astrid Lindgren Children's Hospital, Stockholm, Sweden
Marret Stéphane, Service de Pédiatrie Néonatale et Réanimation, Hôpital Charles Nicolle, Rouen, France
Medja Fadia, INSERM E 9935, Hôpital Robert Debré, Paris, France
Mellier Daniel, Laboratoire de Psychologie et Neurosciences de la Cognition, EA1780, Université de Rouen, Mont-Saint-Aignan, France
Monier Anne, INSERM E 9935 and Service de Neuropédiatrie, Hôpital Robert Debré, Paris, France
Pierrat Véronique, Service de Médecine Néonatale, CHRU de Lille, France
Rattaz Cécile, Service de Médecine Psychologique pour Enfants et Adolescents, CHU Montpellier, France
Rosén Ingmar, Department of Pediatrics and Clinical Neurophysiology, Lund University Hospital, Sweden
Schaal Benoist, Centre des Sciences du Goût, UMR 5170 CNRS-Université de Bourgogne, Dijon, France
Sizun Jacques, Pediatric Department, University Hospital, Brest, France
Soussignan Robert, 2 Unité "Vulnérabilité, Adaptation et Psychopathologie", UMR 7593 CNRS-CHU Salpetrière, Paris, France
Stjernqvist Karin, Dept. of Paediatrics, University of Lund, Lund, Sweden and Dept. of Psychology, University of Lund, Lund, Sweden
Verney Catherine, INSERM E 9935, Hôpital Robert Debré, Paris, France
Warren Inga, Winnicott Baby Unit, St. Mary's Hospital, London, United Kingdom
Westrup Björn, Dept. of Woman and Child Health, Neonatal Programme, Karolinska Institute, Astrid Lindgren Children's Hospital, and Danderyd Hospital, Stockholm, Sweden
Zupan Simunek Véronique, Réanimation néonatale, Hôpital Antoine Béclère, Clamart, France

Contents

Foreword.. VII
    H. Lagercrantz

Part I: Development

- **Brain development in the preterm neonate** 1
  F. Medja, A. Monier, S. Marret, M. Cazillis, C. Verney, P. Gressens

- **Perinatal perceptual development: Some principles derived from psychobiological research**.. 13
  B. Schaal, R. Soussignan, G. Coureaud, D. Mellier

- **Sleep in preterm neonates. Organization, development, deprivation**... 23
  V. Zupan-Simunek, J. Sizun

Part II: Environment

- **Neonatal development: Effects of light**................................. 33
  D. Haumont, V. Hansen

- **Effects of positioning and handling on preterm infants in the neonatal intensive care unit** 39
  K. Bauer

Part III: Developmental care

- **Design and staff issues in light control**.................................. 45
  V. Hansen, D. Haumont

- **Developmental care: A breast-feeding perspective**............... 51
  K. Hedberg Nyqvist

- **Interventions involving positioning and handling in the neonatal intensive care unit: Early developmental care and skin-to-skin holding**... 59
  K. Bauer

- **Non-pharmacological pain control in neonates**.................... 67
  V. Pierrat, N. Goubet, C. Rattaz, T. Debillon

- **The Newborn Individualized Developmental Care and Assessment Program (NIDCAP)** 75
  B. Westrup, A. Kleberg, K. Stjernqvist

- **Implementing developmental care: Considerations for staff** 85
  I. Warren, M. Cuttini

Part IV: Recommendation for research

- **Clinical evaluation of development for research** 93
  C. Amiel-Tison, J. Gosselin

- **Electroencephalography and developmental care** 101
  L. Hellström-Westas, I. Rosén

- **Cerebral Near Infrared Spectroscopy. A useful tool for developmental care research?** 109
  G. Greisen

- **Is it necessary to prove that developmental care is beneficial?** 115
  G. Greisen

- **Points of interest for future research** 119
  H. Lagercrantz, B. Westrup

Foreword

Many more preterm infants survive now than has ever been the case before. They are often products of modern reproductive technology as *in vitro* fertilization. Many of these infants would not survive without treatment with corticosteroids or administration of surfactant and artificial ventilation. The progress of the technical care of the extremely preterm infants has been impressive.

However, the preterm infants are also human beings with consciousness. When they are asleep they are mainly dreaming. When they are awake they respond to sensory stimulation. They react to pain, maybe even more than full term babies, and express emotions.

Regarding the brain the neonatalogists have been mainly concerned with problems like intraventricular haemorrhage and white matter disease. Highly sophisticated techniques have been developed to monitor cerebral blood flow to understand the mechanisms leading to these complications. Less interest has been devoted to the mind and the subjective feelings of the very preterm infant. The research on consciousness is regarded as more airy-fairy and touch-feely questioned by the hard scientists.

The introduction of developmental care by Heidelise Als is a break-through in neonatal care. The importance of this care is that the preterm infant is handled as an individual person with subjective feelings.

Developmental care is now well established in modern neonatology. However, it has taken a long time before it has been accepted by many neonatalogists. The first studies, demonstrating its effects have been heavily attacked mainly on methodological grounds. Although there might have been some methodological problems, the basic idea cannot be questioned any longer. It is paradoxical that more natural methods to handle the very preterm infants such as womb-like care and spontaneous breathing using CPAP evokes such scepticism as compared with much more artificial treatments.

This book summarizes the present state of the art on early developmental care for preterm neonates. We hope this book will be of value for new studies on developmental care.

Hugo Lagercrantz

Acknowledgements

We wish to show our special appreciation to the European Sciences Foundation/European Medical Research Council (ESF/EMRC) that supported our research network on early developmental care for preterm neonates. Special thanks to Mrs Marianne Minkowski and Mrs Carole Moquin-Pattey, Heads of Unit and Senior Scientific Secretaries.

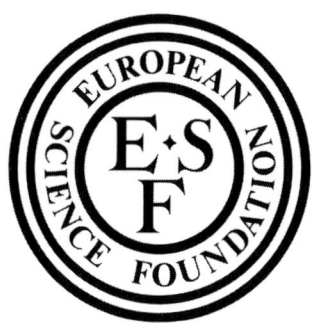

The European Science Foundation (ESF) acts as a catalyst for the development of science by bringing together leading scientists and funding agencies to debate, plan and implement pan-European scientific and science policy initiatives. It is also responsible for the management of COST (European Cooperation in the field of Scientific and Technical Research).

ESF is the European association of 78 major national funding agencies devoted to scientific research in 30 countries. It represents all scientific disciplines: physical and engineering sciences, life, earth and environmental sciences, medical sciences, humanities and social sciences. The Foundation assists its Member Organisations in two main ways. It brings scientists together in its Scientific Forward Looks, Exploratory Workshops, Programmes, Networks, EUROCORES, and ESF Research Conferences, to work on topics of common concern including Research Infrastructures. It also conducts the joint studies of issues of strategic importance in European science policy and manages, on behalf of its Member Organisations, grant schemes, such as EURYI (European Young Investigator Awards).

It maintains close relations with other scientific institutions within and outside Europe. By its activities, the ESF adds value by cooperation and coordination across national frontiers and endeavours, offers expert scientific advice on strategic issues, and provides the European forum for science.

The authors wish to thank Chiesi France Company for their support.

Jacques Sizun is supported by the CNP Foundation.

Brain development in the preterm neonate

Fadia Medja, Anne Monier, Stéphane Marret, Michèle Cazillis, Catherine Verney, Pierre Gressens

Normal development of the human central nervous system (CNS) encompasses several steps including neuroectoderm induction, neurulation, cell proliferation and migration, programmed cell death, neuritogenesis and elimination of excess neurites, synaptogenesis, stabilization and elimination of synapses, gliogenesis and myelination.

These different steps of brain development and maturation are controlled by the interaction between genes and environment. Numerous genes involved in brain development have been identified: genes controlling neurulation, neuronal proliferation, neuronal size and shape, programmed cell death, neuronal-glial interactions, synaptic stabilization [1]. However, it seems unlikely that 30,000 genes in humans can totally control the organization of 100 billions of neurons and trillions of synapses which are involved during development. A normal pattern of expression of these genes requires an adequate environment. Interactions with the intrauterine milieu (factors coming from the mother, placenta, or amniotic fluid) and with the postnatal environment will critically modulate gene expression by interacting with neurotransmitters, trophic factors, hormones or the extracellular matrix.

A central event during brain ontogeny is the migration of neurons from their site of production in the different germinative zones towards their site of function, which can be sometimes located at a distance. In considering neuronal migration, we can divide brain development into three major periods:

1. A premigratory phase covering the period between the individualization of the neural plate and the initiation of neuronal migration;
2. The neuronal migration period;
3. A post-migratory phase, corresponding to the differentiation of neurons which have completed their migration, neuritogenesis, synaptogenesis and the process of stabilisation/elimination.

This chapter will be focused on the neurobiology of events occurring during the post-migratory period, which corresponds in the human neo-cortex, to events observed in the second half of gestation *(figure 1)*. For other steps of brain development, the reader is referred to other review papers [2, 3].

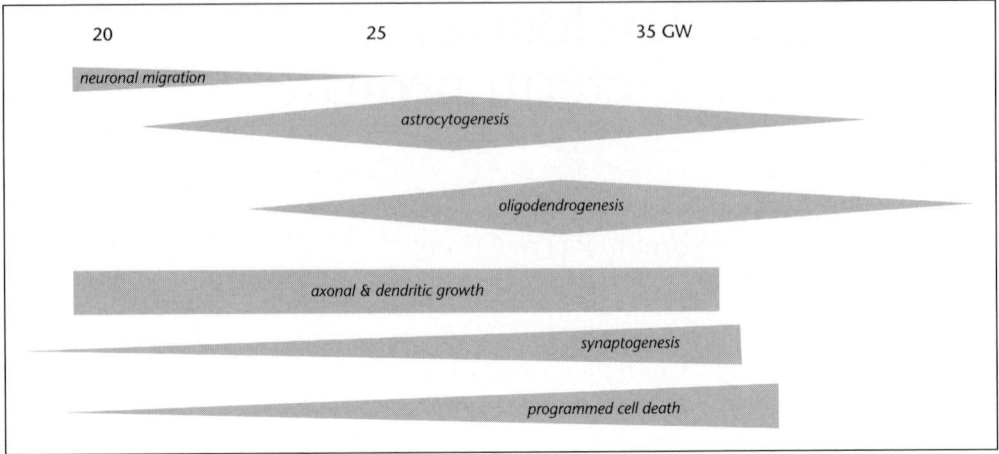

Figure 1. Schematic representation of the major ontogenic events taking place in the human neo-cortex between 20 and 35 gestational weeks (GW).

Neurotransmitters, trophic factors and glucocorticoids

Several neurotransmitters (glutamate, GABA, serotonin, dopamine, catecholamines, different neuropeptides) and trophic factors play important roles at different steps of brain development. It is important to distinguish between the progressive establishment of a neurotransmitter system during brain development in reaching an adult pattern, from the implications these neurotransmitters present in the control or modulation of a specific ontogenic step.

Among neurotransmitters that play a role in brain development, glutamate has been the most characterized. Glutamate is the main excitatory amino acid neurotransmitter in the brain, acting on four main types of receptors: N-methyl-D-aspartate (NMDA), alpha-amino-5-methyl-4-isoxazole propionate (AMPA), kainate and metabotropic receptors. NMDA and AMPA/kainate receptors function as ion channels passing sodium, and under certain circumstances, calcium, whereas metabotropic receptors are G-protein-coupled receptors. In particular, NMDA receptors are particularly involved in the control of neuronal proliferation, migration and survival, axonal growth, and synaptic plasticity.

GABA, which is the main inhibitory neurotransmitter in the adult brain, displays excitatory properties during brain development [4]. For example, in monkeys eight days before birth, it is possible to electrophysiologically record hippocampal neurons which form complex functional networks based on excitatory synapses using GABA as a neurotransmitter [5].

In addition to classical neurotransmitters, several neuropeptides also play important roles during brain development. Vasoactive intestinal peptide (VIP) is a neurotransmitter with modulatory properties in adults but with trophic properties during development. These properties include stimulation of neural stem cell proliferation, modulation of neuronal migration and survival, and stimulation of astrocytogenesis [6]. Interestingly, VIP in rodent and monkey brains, is not detected in large amounts before a stage of brain development corresponding to the third trimester in humans. However, VIP receptors are present very early during brain development. It seems that VIP produced by maternal cells (decidual lymphocytes are good candidates) acts on brain VIP receptors. If these data obtained in animal models can be transposed to the human situation, a very, or extremely preterm human neonate, who loses his/her maternal supply, would have a relative deficit of VIP when compared to a foetus of the same age.

Transmission via the opioid system is by a series of peptide neurotransmitters and hormones, enkephalins, endomorphins, dynorphins. These hormones act on three receptors: mu, beta and kappa receptors. Precursors for some of the peptides (beta-endorphin) are derived from the pro-opiomelanocortin (POMC) gene which is activated in response to stress, and also produces corticocotropin releasing factor (CRF) and hence adrenocorticotrophic hormone, ACTH. Thus there is an important feedback between stress, steroid secretion and opioid function. The functional capacity of the opioid system is increased during pregnancy to mediate spinal analgesia for childbirth, but this system is also partly responsible for the induction of maternal behaviour, at a limbic level [7, 8]. In rhesus monkeys, administration of naloxone reduces maternal affect and grooming [9]. In humans, rejection of the child is more frequent after painful births. Endogenous opioid peptides are also key for the behaviour of the offspring and modulate the early responses to stress and novelty [10]. Thus the opioid system is involved (with glutamate) in defining the set points for glucocorticoid secretion which sets behaviour patterns for the rest of life.

Sub-plate neurons

Sub-plate neurons constitute a distinct structure during neo-cortical development [11]. This structure, localized underneath the neo-cortical plate, reaches its maximal thickness between 22 and 36 gestational weeks.

The first postmitotic neurons produced in the periventricular germinative neuroepithelium will migrate to form a subpial pre-plate or primitive plexiform zone *(figure 2)*. Subsequently produced neurons, which will form the cortical plate, migrate into the pre-plate and split it into the superficial molecular layer (or layer I or marginal zone containing Cajal-Retzius neurons) and the deep sub-plate. Schematically, the successive waves of migratory neurons will pass the sub-plate neurons and end their migratory pathway below layer I, forming successively (but with substantial overlap) cortical layers VI, V, IV, III and II (inside-out pattern). The sub-plate is present in preterm neonates but is not apparent in full-term neonates. Some authors have suggested that these neurons disappear by apoptosis while others have suggested that they are incorporated in layer VI of the mature neo-cortex.

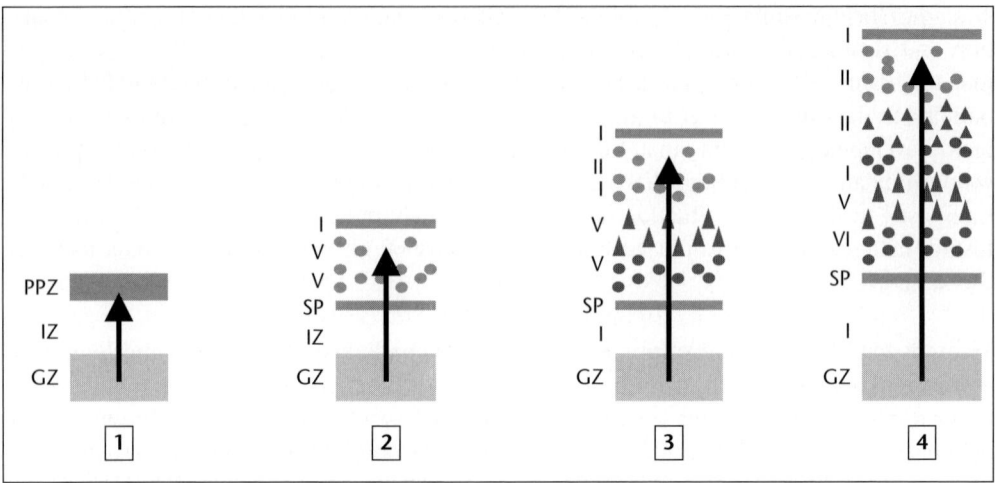

Figure 2. Schematic illustration of mammalian neo-cortical formation. GZ, germinative zone; IZ, intermediate zone (prospective white matter); PPZ, primitive plexiform zone; SP, sub-plate; I, cortical layer I or molecular layer; II to VI, cortical layers II to VI. Arrows and light grey circles indicate migrating neurons while black circles and triangles represent post-migratory neurons.

These sub-plate neurons play several important roles during brain development including:

1. They produce axons for the internal capsule which will serve as guiding axons for axons originating from neurons in layers V and VI;
2. Between 25 and 32 gestational weeks, they produce axons for the corpus callosum;
3. They act as a waiting zone for thalamocortical axons before they invade the cortical plate and reach layer IV.

This waiting zone is necessary for appropriate target selection by thalamocortical afferents. The sub-plate neurons can be lesioned or destroyed in the preterm neonates with periventricular white matter lesions [12]. These data have been recently substantiated in animal models of periventricular white matter damage [13; Husson and Gressens, personal communication].

Programmed cell death

Neurons destined to be in the neo-cortex are produced during the first half of human gestation. Although new neurons can be produced in the dentate gyrus of the hippocampus and in the olfactory bulbs during life, it is generally admitted that, in normal conditions, postnatal and adult neurogenesis is not a key event in the neo-cortex [14]. Therefore, during normal brain development, neuronal production in the neo-cortex is largely completed by the time very or extremely preterm neonates are born. This also true for migration of neo-cortical neurons which ends at around 24 weeks of gestation.

However, this neuronal equipment is not fixed. Between 15 and 50 per cent, according to brain areas, of the initially formed neurons will be eliminated by a physiological process called programmed cell death or apoptosis. About 70% of these neurons which are destined to disappear, seem to die between 28 and 41 gestational weeks [15]. This programmed cell death is a complex mechanism that involves a balance between death and trophic signals, death and survival genetic programs, and effectors and inhibitors of cell death [16].

Electrical activity seems to be a critical factor for neuronal survival. In rodents, administration of drugs which block electrical activity during the period of brain growth spurt, leads to a dramatic exacerbation of neuronal cell death in different brain areas. These drugs include NMDA receptor blockers (MK-801 or ketamine), GABA-A receptor agonists such as classical antiepileptic drugs (phenytoin, phenobarbital, diazepam, clonazepam, vigabatrin, or valproic acid) and anaesthetics (combination of midazolam, nitrous oxide, and isoflurane) [17, 18]. These effects on neuronal cell death are mimicked by acute administration of ethanol, blocking NMDA receptors and activating GABA-A receptors [19]. Although the mechanism is unknown, the systemic injection to newborn mouse pups of a combination of sulfites (which are present in the excipient of some commercially available preparation of injectable glucocorticoids and vasoactive amines) and dexamethasone, lead to an exacerbation of programmed neural cell death both in the neocortex and in basal ganglia [20].

Axons and dendrites

When neurons are reaching their final destination, they start to produce axons and dendrites, allowing connection of distant cerebral structures. This ontogenic step is occurring largely, but not exclusively, during the second half of gestation and extends into the postnatal period. For example, evoked visual potentials can be produced as early as 24-27 gestational weeks in human neonates, confirming the existence of an established wiring at this early developmental stage [21].

During brain development, axonal growth cones, which are located at the tip of the growing axon, must find their way through the maturating brain structures to reach their target. Different mechanisms play a role in the path finding process, including chemoattraction and chemorepulsion, release of neurotransmitter and trophic factors, interactions with the extracellular matrix, and guidance by pioneer axons which connected brain structures at early stages of development when distances were not as great.

Some of the connections between brain structures are highly controlled by genetic programs and are marginally influenced by experience, while other types of connections (such as corpus callosum fibers, for example) are much more susceptible to environmental factors acting during the uterine and postnatal life. The interaction between genetic programs and environmental stimuli lead to the maintenance of some connections and the elimination of other aberrant or redundant connections.

Synapses

Synaptogenesis is a process of excess production followed by elimination of some synapses, and strengthening or stabilization of others. This ontogenic step is initiated in the neo-cortex at mid-gestation, with a peak during the two first postnatal years, and which ends at puberty [22, 23]. Changeux and Danchin [24] and Edelman [25] have proposed the concept of synaptic stabilization (with the elimination of not stabilized synapses). In a schematic way, during brain development there are successive waves of overproduction of labile synapses, inducing redundant connections produced in a relatively random manner. This step is under tight genetic control. Each wave of overproduction is followed by a period of stabilization of synapses that have a functional meaning, and elimination of those that are redundant or meaningless. This period of stabilization and elimination is highly influenced by environmental stimuli and experience. NMDA receptors, NO°, neuronal depolarization and competition for trophic factors are among key factors controlling this stabilization-elimination process [26, 27].

Astrocytes

Glia is composed of three types of cells: astrocytes, oligodendrocytes and microglia (brain macrophages). Neo-cortical astrocytes have a dual origin [28]:

1. After the end of neuronal migration, radial glial cells (which are glial cells specialized in the guidance of migrating neurons) transform into astrocytes which are found mainly in the deep cortical layers and underlying white matter;
and 2. The periventricular germinative zone produces, after the end of neuronal production, astrocytic precursors, which will migrate mostly into the superficial neo-cortical layers.

In humans, this astrocytic proliferation probably takes place between 24 and 32 weeks of gestation, with a peak around 26 weeks. This might be particularly important for preterm neonates. Indeed, astrocytes play several important roles including axonal guidance, stimulation of neuritic growth, transfer of metabolites between blood vessels and neurons, establishment of scaffolding structures, production of extracellular matrix components, production of trophic factors, and participation in the functioning of the blood-brain-barrier. Experimentally, blockading of VIP receptors at a stage corresponding to preterm delivery (mimicking the potential VIP deficiency of human preterm neonates – see above) leads to a transient but significant reduction of the astrocytic density in the neo-cortex [29]. This transient astrocytic depletion is accompanied by an increased neuronal programmed cell death and long-term changes in neo-cortical synaptic structure [30].

Oligodendrocytes and myelination

Myelination occurs during a protracted period, ending long after birth. Although myelination leads to a marked acceleration of nerve conduction, human and experimental studies have reported several examples of dissociation between the degree of myelination and the maturation of a given function.

Oligodendrocytes, which produce myelin, can be divided into four cell types according to their stage of maturation: progenitors, late progenitors, immature oligodendrocytes and mature oligodendrocytes. The second type is the dominant cell type in the second half of gestation in the periventricular white matter. These late progenitors are highly vulnerable to oxidative stress, excitotoxic cascade (through AMPA-kainate receptors) and hypoxic-ischemic insults during the pre-myelination period (extending roughly until 32 weeks of gestation) [31, 32, 33].

Microglia

Microglia constitute 5-15 per cent of the total cerebral cellular population. The prevailing view is that microglia are derived from circulating precursors in blood, which originate from bone marrow [34, 35]. During the first trimester of human gestation penetrating cells have an amoeboid morphology with large ovoid cell bodies and no or few short processes. These cells express macrophage antigenic characteristics depending on their location and activation state [36]. This macrophagic morphology evolved in intermediate and mature phenotypes with a smaller cell body and longer processes [37]. At mid-gestation macrophages-microglia populations are mostly detected within the white matter pathways as the external and internal capsules and corpus callosum [38]. As suggested from rodent studies these cells could contribute to the physiological developmental remodelling: phagocytosis of cellular fragments produced by neuro-developmental apoptosis and elimination of exuberant axons and dendrites [39, 40]. However, the correlation between regressive events and the distribution of macrophages is not clear, suggesting other possible functions during development [41]. In the case of cerebral lesions, some authors suggest a possible neurotoxic role of the cerebral macrophage in the production of free radicals and nitrite oxyde [41]. Under pathological conditions, microglial cells can be activated in functional brain macrophages with reappearance of specific cell surface markers. Following development, mature microglia constitute a quiescent cellular population with small cell bodies and numerous long, thin processes. They may play a role in regulation of the extracellular environment and immune protection of the brain.

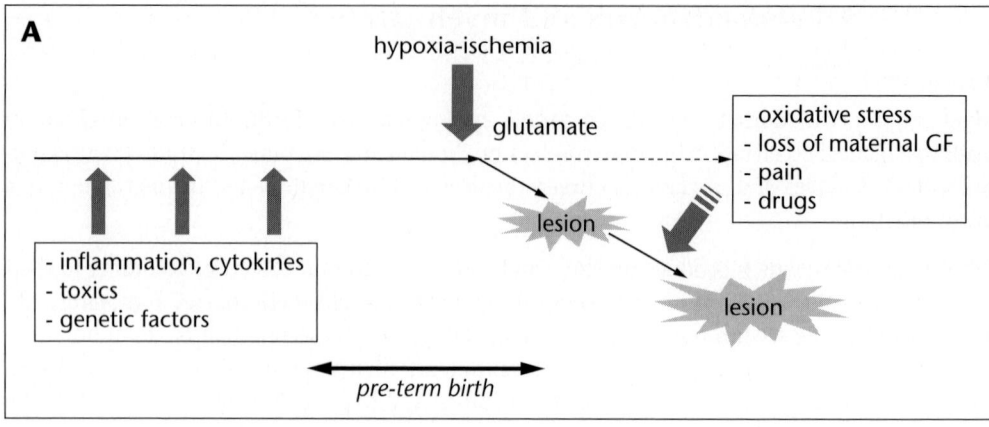
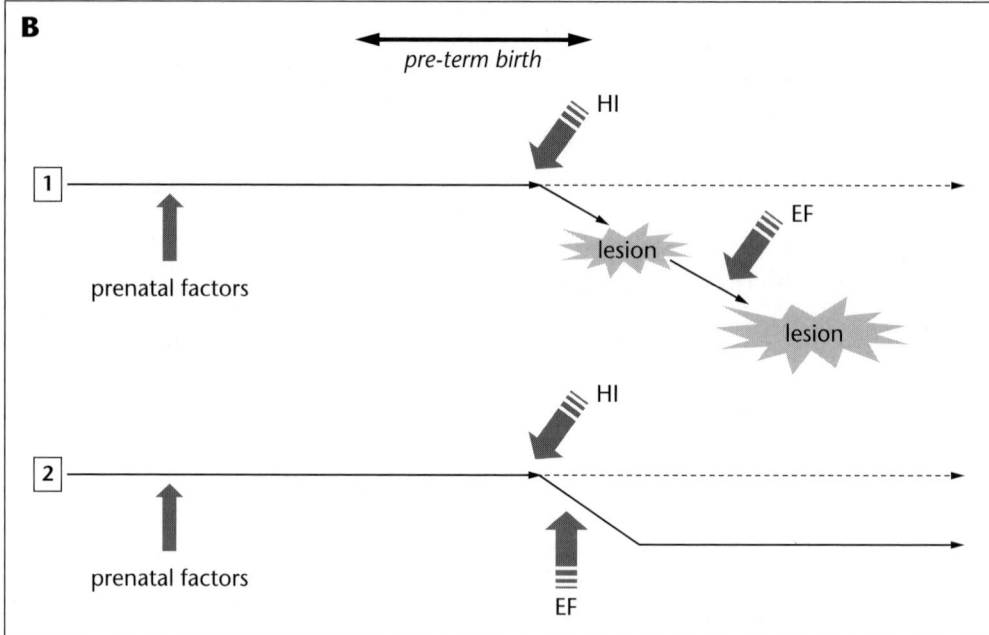

Figure 3. A. Schematic representation of the pathophysiology of clastic brain lesions (GF = growth factors). **B.** Comparison of the pathophysiological hypotheses underlying clastic brain lesions (1) and non-clastic brain impairments (2) (HI = hypoxia-ischemia; EF = environmental factor).

Conclusions

In order to get a better understanding of the pathophysiology of brain disturbances underlying neuropsychological impairments in preterm neonates, brain development has to be considered both in its cytoarchitectonic and its physiological dimensions. One largely unexplored field is the impact of the *ex utero* environment of a preterm neonate on brain development and maturation when compared to the *in utero* situation.

Preterm and very preterm infants are at risk for the development of destructive (clastic) brain lesions such as periventricular leukomalacia which can be detected on brain imaging (sonograms and MRI), and which are responsible for motor and cognitive sequellae [42]. The pathophysiology of these clastic lesions is likely multifactorial, including hypoxic-ischemic conditions, excess release of glutamate (leading to the excitotoxic cascade), inflammatory factors such as cytokines, oxidative stress, growth factor deficiency, genes of susceptibility or resistance, exposure to toxins (including drugs), maternal stress, or pain and other excessive stimuli *(figure 3A)*.

In contrast, extremely preterm infants rarely develop clastic brain lesions although they are at very high risk to develop neurological, motor and cognitive defects [43, 44]. This suggests that other mechanisms are operating in order to alter genetic programs of brain development, inducing long-lasting disturbances of specific neuronal networks. We can propose the hypothesis that some of the above-mentioned factors could also disturb some steps of brain development (such as programmed neuronal death, neuronal differentiation, astrocytogenesis or oligodendrogenesis) without inducing clastic lesions. This may occur when they act at a more immature stage of brain development with less severe intensity *(figure 3B)*.

References

1. Simeone A. Towards the comprehension of genetic mechanisms controlling brain morphogenesis. *Trends Neurosci* 2002; 25: 119-21.

2. Caviness VS, Takahashi T, Nowakowski RS. Morphogenesis of the human cerebral cortex. In: Peter G Barth, ed. *Disorders of neuronal migration*. England: Mac Keith Press, 2003: 1-23.

3. Gressens P. Neuronal migration. In: Lagercrantz H, Evrard P, Hanson M, Rodeck C, eds. *The newborn brain: scientific basis and clinical applications*. Cambridge University Press, 2001: 69-90.

4. Ben-Ari Y, Khazipov R, Leinekugel X, Caillard O, Gaiarsa JL. GABAA, NMDA and AMPA receptors: a developmentally regulated "menage a trois". *Trends Neurosci* 1997; 20: 523-9.

5. Khazipov R, Esclapez M, Caillard O, *et al*. Early development of neuronal activity in the primate hippocampus in utero. *J Neurosci* 2001; 21: 9770-81.

6. Brenneman DE, Hill JM, Gressens P, Gozes I. Neurotrophic action of VIP: from CNS ontogeny to therapeutic strategy. In: Said SS, ed. *Pro-inflammatory and anti-inflammatory peptides*. M. Dekker, Inc, New York, 1997: 383-408.

7. Mann DR, Orr TE. Effect of restraint stress on gonadal pro-opiomelanocortin peptides and the pituitary-testicular axis in rats. *Life Sci* 1990; 46: 1601-9.

8. Panksepp J, Nelson E, Siviy S. Brain opioids and mother-infant social motivation. *Acta Paediatr Suppl* 1994; 397: 40-6.

9. Martel FL, Nevison CM, Rayment FD, Simpson MJ, Keverne EB. Opioid receptor blockade reduces maternal affect and social grooming in rhesus monkeys. *Psychoneuroendocrinology* 1993; 18: 307-21.

10. Martel FL, Nevison CM, Simpson MJ, Keverne EB. Effects of opioid receptor blockade on the social behavior of rhesus monkeys living in large family groups. *Dev Psychobiol* 1995; 28: 71-84.

11. Kostovic I, Judas M. Correlation between the sequential ingrowth of afferents and transient patterns of cortical lamination in preterm infants. *Anat Rec* 2002; 267: 1-6.

12. Sarnat HB, Flores-Sarnat L. A new classification of malformations of the nervous system: an integration of morphological and molecular genetic criteria as patterns of genetic expression. *Eur J Paediatr Neurol* 2001; 5: 57-64.

13. McQuillen PS, Sheldon RA, Shatz CJ, Ferriero DM. Selective vulnerability of subplate neurons after early neonatal hypoxia-ischemia. *J Neurosci* 2003; 23: 3308-15.

14. Taupin P, Gage FH. Adult neurogenesis and neural stem cells of the central nervous system in mammals. *J Neurosci Res* 2002; 69: 745-9.

15. Bhutta AT, Anand KJ. Abnormal cognition and behavior in preterm neonates linked to smaller brain volumes. *Trends Neurosci* 2001; 24: 129-30; discussion 131-2.

16. Vaudry D, Falluel-Morel A, Leuillet S, Vaudry H, Gonzalez BJ. Regulators of cerebellar granule cell development act through specific signaling pathways. *Science* 2003; 300: 1532-4.

17. Bittigau P, Sifringer M, Genz K, et al. Antiepileptic drugs and apoptotic neurodegeneration in the developing brain. *Proc Natl Acad Sci USA* 2002; 99: 15089-94.

18. Jevtovic-Todorovic V, Hartman RE, Izumi Y, et al. Early exposure to common anesthetic agents causes widespread neurodegeneration in the developing rat brain and persistent learning deficits. *J Neurosci* 2003; 23: 876-82.

19. Ikonomidou C, Bittigau P, Ishimaru MJ, et al. Ethanol-induced apoptotic neurodegeneration and fetal alcohol syndrome. *Science* 2000; 287: 1056-60.

20. Baud O. Is perinatal dexamethasone treatment safe in preterm infants? *Dev Med Child Neurol Suppl* 2001; 86: 23-5.

21. Tabary JC. Faut-il conserver la notion de maturation du SNC. *Motricité cérébrale* 2002, 23: 7-19.

22. Garner CC, Zhai RG, Gundelfinger ED, Ziv NE. Molecular mechanisms of CNS synaptogenesis. *Trends Neurosci* 2002; 25: 243-51.

23. Bourgeois JP. Synaptogenesis, heterochrony and epigenesis in the mammalian neo-cortex. *Acta Paediatr Suppl* 1997; 422: 27-33.

24. Changeux JP, Danchin A. Selective stabilisation of developing synapses as a mechanism for the specification of neuronal networks. *Nature* 1976; 264: 705-12.

25. Edelman GM. Group selection as the basis for higher brain function. In: Schmitt FO, Worden FC, Adelman G, Dennis SG, eds. *The organisation of cerebral cortex*. Cambridge: MIT Press, 1981: 535-63.

26. Gan WB, Kwon E, Feng G, Sanes JR, Lichtman JW. Synaptic dynamism measured over minutes to months: age-dependent decline in an autonomic ganglion. *Nat Neurosci* 2003; 6: 956-60.

27. Nelson PG, Jia M, Li MX. Protein kinases and Hebbian function. *Neuroscientist* 2003; 9: 110-6.

28. Gressens P, Richelme C, Kadhim HJ, Gadisseux JF, Evrard P. The germinative zone produces the most cortical astrocytes after neuronal migration in the developing mammalian brain. *Biol Neonate* 1992; 61: 4-24.

29. Zupan V, Hill JM, Brenneman DE, et al. Involvement of pituitary adenylate cyclase-activating polypeptide II vasoactive intestinal peptide 2 receptor in mouse neo-cortical astrocytogenesis. *J Neurochem* 1998; 70: 2165-73.

30. Zupan V, Nehlig A, Evrard P, Gressens P. Prenatal blockade of vasoactive intestinal peptide alters cell death and synaptic equipment in the murine neo-cortex. *Pediatr Res* 2000; 47: 53-63.

31. Follett PL, Rosenberg PA, Volpe JJ, Jensen FE. NBQX attenuates excitotoxic injury in developing white matter. *J Neurosci* 2000; 20: 9235-41.

32. Back SA, Han BH, Luo NL, *et al.* Selective vulnerability of late oligodendrocyte progenitors to hypoxia-ischemia. *J Neurosci* 2002; 22: 455-63.

33. Haynes RL, Folkerth RD, Keefe RJ, *et al.* Nitrosative and oxidative injury to premyelinating oligodendrocytes in periventricular leukomalacia. *J Neuropathol Exp Neurol* 2003; 62: 441-50.

34. Ling EA, Wong WC. The origin and nature of ramified and amoeboid microglia: a historical review and current concepts. *Glia* 1993; 7: 9-18.

35. Perry VH, Gordon S. Macrophages and microglia in the nervous system. *Trends Neurosci* 1988; 11: 273-7.

36. Andjelkovic AV, Nikolic B, Pachter JS, Zecevic N. Macrophages/microglial cells in human central nervous system during development: an immunohistochemical study. *Brain Res* 1998; 814: 13-25.

37. Rezaie P, Male D. Colonisation of the developing human brain and spinal cord by microglia: a review. *Microsc Res Tech* 1999; 45: 359-82.

38. Gould SJ, Howard S. An immunohistological study of macrophages in the human fetal brain. *Neuropathol Appl Neurobiol* 1991; 17: 383-90.

39. Innocenti GM, Koppel H, Clarke S. Transitory macrophages in the white matter of the developing visual cortex. I. Light and electron microscopic characteristics and distribution. *Brain Res* 1983; 313: 39-53.

40. Innocenti GM, Clarke S, Koppel H. Transitory macrophages in the white matter of the developing visual cortex. II. Development and relations with axonal pathways. *Brain Res* 1983; 313: 55-66.

41. Mallat M, Chamak B. Brain macrophages: neurotoxic or neurotrophic effector cells? *J Leukoc Biol* 1994; 56: 416-22.

42. Volpe JJ. Neurobiology of periventricular leukomalacia in the premature infant. *Pediat Res* 2001; 50: 553-62.

43. Luoma L, Herrgard E, Martikainen A. Neuropsychological analysis of the visuomotor problems in children born preterm at < or = 32 weeks of gestation: a 5-year prospective follow-up. *Dev Med Child Neurol* 1998; 40: 21-30.

44. Luoma L, Herrgard E, Martikainen A, Ahonen T. Speech and language development of children born at < or = 32 weeks' gestation: a 5-year prospective follow-up study. *Dev Med Child Neurol* 1998; 40: 380-7.

Perinatal perceptual development: Some principles derived from psychobiological research

Benoist Schaal, Robert Soussignan, Gérard Coureaud, Daniel Mellier

This chapter deals with several principles derived from psychobiological research on the development of perceptual and behavioural processes in mammalian foetuses and newborns. It aims to sum up some strategies evolved by the brain to cope with species-specific constraints to which perinatal organisms are exposed during normal transitions of life, and how these strategies may be challenged in the case of atypical life transitions (*e.g.*, mother-infant separation for long duration, premature birth).

Some principles of sensory development

Phylogenetic legacy

A first general principle is that not only the structural and functional properties of sensory systems (what and how they perceive) but also the pace of their relative development (when they begin to perceive) are an outcome of natural history. Sensory systems are thus designed to respond to a given set of stimuli at given times in ontogeny to adaptively sustain the organism in the face of normal challenges raised by the species-typical course of development. This principle underscores that the perceptual abilities of perinatal organisms are the end-point of evolved strategies of which contemporary care practitioners may be usefully informed. Additionally, it calls attention to the value of taking into account research conducted in various animal models to enlarge and update knowledge that may have theoretical validity and practical applicability for the care of human foetuses, newborns and infants.

Immature, but adapted sensory functions

A second principle is that, despite structural and functional immaturity, all sensory systems in foetal and neonatal organisms are more or less reactive to the stimuli they are devised to process.

In addition, not only do these systems sense the perinatal environments, but they also extract meaningful information that is stored in neural networks and memory for variable durations. Attempts have been made to identify times of development of sensory, and eventually, integrative abilities in foetuses and newborns. However, these time-points may be at best indicative rather than absolute because of the variable conditions in which investigations have been conducted [see ref 1, 2 for recent reviews on the foetal agenda of sensory development]. In our own species, all sensory systems are at least partially active in the last trimester of gestation, and functionally nearly similar in the last-month foetus and in the newborn (perhaps at the exception of vision). These sensory systems have all been demonstrated to derive information from the prenatal ecological niche and to transfer it into the postnatal niche [for reviews on the different sensory modalities, see ref 3, 4]. The sensory awareness of the foetus is thus at the start of a general phenomenon of transnatal perceptual continuity which potential contribution to the adaptive responsiveness of the newborn should not be overlooked in clinical context (see below).

Time-order of sensory onsets

With ongoing foetal research, the exact dates for our understanding of sensory onset are subject to change. It seems certain, however, that the relative timing of sensory inception is constant in amniotes. This constitutes a third principle, which states that sensory development starts along a non-random sequence among the different sensory modalities. Specifically, somesthesic processes are identified earliest in development, closely followed by chemosensory, kinesthetic and auditory processes and, lastly, proceeding to visual capacities [5]. The corollary of this sequential sensory onset is the sequential "opening" of the brain to sensory experience. This has been viewed [6] as a strategy to reduce the nature, amount and complexity of stimulation available to maturing neural tissue and to regulate the competition between emerging sensory modalities. It is to be noted that the proximoceptive modalities (touch, kinesthesis, chemoreception) normally develop earlier than the teloceptive modalities (hearing, vision). It may be anticipated that altering the inborn ordering between earlier developing senses and later developing senses (either by experimental provision of stimulations before normal time or by preterm birth) may modify the evolved limitation of sensory input to the brain and thereby modify the perceptual organisation in the organism. This has been amply documented in animal perinates [*e.g.*, 7, 8]. For example, rat pups (born with eyes closed until day 14) provided earlier-than-normal visual stimulation exhibit accelerated visual responsiveness, but a deterioration in their usual reliance on olfactory cues in an orientation task [9]. Much alike, quail embryos receiving abnormally early visual input show accelerated visual preference to maternal visual gestalt, but express decline in their normal response to maternal auditory cues [10]. Such intersensory effects remain to be understood in human perinates.

Specialisation through developmental heterochrony

A fourth principle, which refines the previous one, is that within each of the functioning modalities the maturation of sensory and corresponding neuromotor processes appear to be heterogeneous in topography and timing. That is, the local maturation of the various sensors within a modality appears to anticipate processes that will be recruited in the subsequent developmental niche. For example, it is noteworthy in the late-gestation foetus that tactile terminals undergo advanced maturation in the oral and perioral fields and are coupled with directional actions of the head [*e.g.*, 11, 12]. Tactile endings also differentiate sooner on the fingers and palms than on the rest of the body. Contact between these body parts richly endowed with tactile sensors (lip-lip, finger-tongue, hand-mouth, hand-hand) initiate various motor actions in perinates, which support the stimulation of haptic pathways and contribute to organise oral activities (licking, sucking). Chemosensory development concurs as well to the modulation of future oral actions and appears to be biased towards the detection of certain stimuli that are to be encountered in the next developmental niche. For example, the milk of the species seems to be more potent than the milk of another species in releasing appetitive and ingestive responses for late gestation foetuses and ingestion-naïve newborns. This chemosensory bias towards compounds from homospecific milk has been documented in several mammals, including our own [*e.g.*, 13, 14]. However, the nature of the stimuli, as well as the neural pathways involved, remain generally unidentified. These examples illustrate that besides the mainstream development of sensory systems, specialisations in specific sensory capacities can arise from local differentiation phenomena which are quantitatively or qualitatively disparate.

Experience-dependent plasticity

The fifth principle is that neurosensory structures and their functional performances are facilitated or organized through experience within the individual-specific environment. One of the most notable achievements of contemporary neuroscience show how sensory macro-organisation is under experience-independent processes, and how the fine-tuning (through neuronal selection, inter-neuronal connectivity) of the sensory organs, connecting centres and corresponding motor loops are tightly dependent on sensory impact [*e.g.*, 15, 16, 17]. Experiments using sensory deprivation, selective enrichment of the environment, or surgical decoupling of sensory structures from centres have shown that all sensory modalities are susceptible to such environmental influences during either prenatal or early postnatal development. These epigenetic influences are most potent during certain phases of neurosensory ontogeny, so called "sensitive periods", when they have the ability to imprint more or less definitively the subsequent perceptual profile of the organism. Any functional deficit can eventually be recuperated by supplemental or compensatory stimulation if it intervenes before the "closure" of the corresponding sensitive period. Although research on experience-dependent plasticity has mainly been concerned with intramodal processes, as mentioned above, the articulation between modalities and intermodal integration are also largely dependent on experience.

It ensues from these five principles that early sensory, cognitive and behavioural development is the selected end-point of multi-determined, interactive, temporally-ordered processes. The final properties of organisms are prevalently canalised by experience. Some perceptual specialisations may emerge uninfluenced (or minimally influenced) by experience ("predispositions", see below), however, making the newborn organism simultaneously a perceptual specialist attending to particular stimuli and a skilful generalist prone to react to and learn any stimulus linked with beneficial (or detrimental) effects in the environment. Perceptual development is time-ordered, both within and between sensory modalities, in a way that the sensory assemblies "cooperate" towards the production of neural representations which direct neonatal actions in the normal postnatal mother-infant context.

The formation of perceptual expectations in foetuses and newborns

Newborn infants do not orient randomly to sensory stimuli after birth. Some stimuli are more efficient than others in releasing interest and approach. Understanding the origin and causes of the perceptual efficiency of the stimuli world into which newborns are immersed, and how newborns sort out meaningful stimuli from the environment has been the topic of a considerable amount of study and theorizing [*e.g.*, 18, 19, 20]. As a rule, newborns show preferential attention and responses to stimuli with which they have previously become familiar, or for which they bear a predisposed perceptual structure.

Sensory experience in an earlier developmental context may create "perceptual expectations" towards those objects bearing similar sensory features in subsequent contexts. Sensory expectations based on prior experience have been abundantly described in mammalian newborns. For example, neonatal responses influenced by exposure to sounds or odours during the embryonic/foetal period have been documented in various birds and mammals [*cf.* reviews in 21, 22, 23]. Such prenatally acquired perceptual expectations have been shown in term-born human infants as well. Foetuses acquire some voice or speech-relevant cues afforded by their mother, and newborns are attentive to them. These responses have been demonstrated by the neonatal propensity to "work" by sucking on a non-nutritive nipple to obtain the play-back of a tape-recording of their mother's voice [24]; intrauterine physiological noises [25]; or a rhyme repeatedly uttered by the mother during pregnancy [26]. The neonatal auditory system can thus pick out cues from the postnatal sound environment which have been prenatally endowed with reinforcing potency. Likewise, human newborns exhibit preferential orientation to an odour they have experienced in the womb during the last weeks of pregnancy [27, 28]. Finally, some these also reveal neonatal expectations in terms of stimulation intensity. Soft "social" touch as opposed to the more sturdy clinical touch has been shown to affect postnatal growth of premature newborns [29, 30].

After birth, newborns expand the variety and range of their sensory expectations as a function of their experiences in their individual environment. For example, newborns exposed to repeated stroking of the forehead followed by the delivery of sucrose rapidly show appetitive responses upon being simply stroked [31], thus indicating the establishment of a regularity in stroking-taste association. When this regularity is violated by uncoupling the sucrose administration from the stroking, the infants' appetitive responses diminish rapidly (in only two sessions) in the same time that emotionally negative responses (negative faces, crying) increase. Thus, human newborns create expectations among contingent or sequential events from the first hours or days after birth [32].

Finally, in some cases, neonatal sensory expectations have been shown to develop in the absence of previous experience. For example, newly born rabbits evince a very robust response to an odorant carried in rabbit milk without prenatal nor postnatal exposure to it [14]. In humans, newborn infants prefer from birth to look at a schematic face rather than at a scrambled face [33]. It has been suggested that this visually-guided orientation towards the human face derives from a predisposed perceptual process [34, 35].

In sum, infant expectations for given stimuli may rely on a variety of nonexclusive mechanisms ranging from genetically transmitted stimulus-response coupling to opportunistic learning in the earliest stages of development.

Perinatal sensory continuity and some effects of imposed discontinuity

The late-gestation foetus and the newborn's formation of sensory expectations contributes to a tendency to screen out corresponding stimuli and lays the groundwork for relative continuity from before to after birth. This transnatal continuity in perception is paralleled with an overlap in the sensory properties of the both perinatal environments [36]. All conditions are present in both environments for the newly born infant to effectively use the prenatally acquired information. These perceptual and ecological components of the transnatal sensory continuity hypotheses have been directly tested with both sounds and odours. The above mentioned work by DeCasper and colleagues has conclusively demonstrated continuity effects from foetal auditory experience to neonatal preferences for certain sounds. Such effects can arise in normal life conditions where a given tune is associated with relaxed states of the pregnant mother, and can contribute to calming in the newborn [37, 38]. In the olfactory modality, investigations mentioned above have established the selective retention of prenatally-acquired odour sensations in neonates. Other studies simultaneously exposed 3-day old newborns to stimuli they were exposed to before birth, amniotic fluid, and to a stimulus they were never exposed to, their mother's colostrum. The newborns oriented their nose equally to both stimuli [39], leading to the hypothesis that they perceived both as sensorily or motivationally equivalent. Similar outcomes were reached in various mammalian newborns [36, for review], providing additional support for the notion of a relative continuity in both perinatal odour environments and perceptual abilities.

If perinatal sensory continuity has an adaptive meaning, its experimental disruption should have measurable consequences, but few experiments have examined this phenomenon. The consequences of violating olfactory expectations established *in utero* were examined by introducing prematurely delivered rat pups into warmed containers varying in odour atmospheres [40]. Four groups of pups were put for the first postnatal hour into warmed containers scented with either 1. Amniotic odour, 2. An odorant which is present in maternal saliva, 3. A novel odour (mint) and 4. Nothing (control). Whereas the control, amniotic, and maternal odour groups showed more than 80% of viable animals, the novel odor group evinced only 50% of surviving pups. For premature rats, being introduced into an odorised atmosphere that bears no sensory link with the prenatal environment has clear detrimental effects.

Relying on a less dramatic alteration of the olfactory environment, another study compared the response of rabbit newborns exposed to perinatal odour continuity or discontinuity [41]. Immediately after term delivery, half of each litter was fostered to a female that had eaten the same diet as their biological mother, the other half were housed with a female that had eaten an olfactory-different diet. In this way, a group of "continuous" pups (*i.e.*, exposed to perinatal continuity) and a group of "discontinuous" pups were obtained. Both groups of pups were followed during the first 3 suckling opportunities for sucking success and amount of milk consumed[1]. The "continuous" pups demonstrated a better sucking, and ingested more milk than the "discontinuous" pups in the first two suckling bouts. Moreover, an additional experiment which exposed newborns to milk samples carrying the dominant odor of the diet consumed by their mother during gestation. The newborn rabbits were more attracted to the milk that was olfactorily matched with their foetal experience [41]. Thus, the condition in which the olfactory properties of the mother's belly or milk are consistent with olfactory expectations acquired *in utero* determines more efficient searching and sucking performance in rabbit neonates.

Interference with transnatal olfactory continuity may be expected in the practice of feeding infants with formulae of heterospecific (bovine or vegetal) origin. Breast- and bottle-fed infants can be seen as exposed perinatally to continuous and discontinuous odour environments, respectively. When infants from either category are simultaneously presented with the odours of their own mother's amniotic fluid and of the milk they have been introduced to, their pattern of response differs markedly over postnatal days 2 to 4. The response of breast-fed infants changes from nondiscrimination on day 2 to the expression of a clear preference for the breast milk odour over the amniotic odour on day 4 [42]. In the same conditions, exclusively bottle-fed infants exhibit a clear response in favour of the amniotic odour on day 2 and maintain this preferential orientation on day 4 [43]. In other words, when facing the odours of two biologically relevant substrates experienced pre- and postnatally, breast-fed infants develop a preference for the breast milk relatively quickly, while bottle-fed infants remain more attracted to the prenatal odour than to the odour to which they were exposed postnatally 6 times a day for 4 days. Although multiple rationale may be contemplated in this subtle differential development of odor preferences, the impact of the disruption in transnatal chemosensory continuity cannot be ruled out.

From the above discussion, one may hypothesise that a transition which is matched, as opposed to a transition which is not matched, with an olfactory expectation derived from previous experience may lead to a differential engagement of positive responsiveness. These responses may be demonstrated by behavioural approach tendencies, nutritional intake, and readiness to learn. These results emphasize the importance of sensory expectations acquired in the foetus and used

---

1. Rabbit females suckle their pups once per day for only 5 minutes, so that missing two consecutive sucking opportunities seriously jeopardises outcomes.

by the newborn to adaptively bridge the birth transition. However, a variety of events and contexts may lead to the further establishment of olfactory expectations during later phases of development. Among those, familiarization as well as various reinforcing processes (*e.g.*, satiation, comfort contact) must be considered. Thus, the above logic is not restricted to the birth transition, but can be applied to every transition occurring later in typical (*e.g.*, weaning, "adoption" of new life settings or caring persons) or atypical development (*e.g.*, introduction into an incubator, transition from tube to bottle- or to breast-feeding).

Clinical prospects

The above discussion demonstrates that the external stimuli that have become sensorily or motivationally salient during prenatal/postnatal development can be reliably identified through the behavioural and physiological responses of the foetus/neonate. An infant's sensory expectations can be functionally gauged by various responses ranging from psychophysiological changes, distress attenuation, elicitation of positive orientation and active approach, to the optimisation of metabolic processes. Such infant response-based approaches have often been used to assess sensory preferences in term-born infants, but more rarely in premature infants. Notable exceptions are the preterm infants' *active* approach of objects bearing soft and warm tactile properties as well as rhythmic stimulation [*e.g.*, 44], facilitated energy conservation through the application of tactile stimulation [*e.g.*, 29, 45], beneficial physiological and behavioural consequences of the infant's direct contact with the mother's skin [*e.g.*, 46, 47], and the calming effects of sweet taste [*e.g.*, 48]. These are some prominent findings that are currently being progressively incorporated into care practices [see 49, for review].

Similar data may be derived from analysing the species-typical system of interactions between the growing organism and their environment in the foetal and early postnatal periods. A detailed characterization of 1. The sensory ecology in which infants typically develop *in* and *ex utero*, and of 2. Their abilities to perceive, recognize and react to these sensory cues may identify sensory invariants of the original environments, as well as the sources of individual variability. Such normative knowledge may serve as reference to guide the formulation of the sensory (physical and social) environment of infants undergoing atypical trajectories of development (*e.g.*, preterm birth; term born but postnatally separated from the mother). The same quantitative approach should be used to depict the artificial niches into which such infants are raised, so that their departure from the original expected ecological niches can be reduced. Such an approach is further advocated by Heidelise Als [50].

We are aware that the facts gathered from *in utero* foetuses and term newborns are to be transposed cautiously to preterm infants who represent heterogeneous populations and are developing along fluctuating rules [51]. Examples may be derived from studies on infant stress and pain responses. While preterm infants are more reactive (skin conductance response) than term infants to being carried, or to position change, they are paradoxically less reactive to heel prick [52]. Further, fewer facial emotional responses measured by infrared thermography when exposed to a pure odorant in 32-34 week-old infants (gestational age) than in younger (30-31 weeks) or older (> 35 weeks) infants [53]. In the foetus [54], the mechanisms underlying such developmental fluctuations are not well understood.

Finally, the scientific enquiry of perceptual development has not followed the ordered timing of sensory input. Earlier emerging sensory modalities of proximal senses (such as touch, chemoreception, and pain) have not been studied to the extent that later-developing, distal senses (audition, vision) have. This trend of knowledge acquisition, based on an adultocentric perspective of infant sensory development, has no link with the adaptive importance of the senses in neonatal behaviour. It reveals that the functional status of certain sensory systems (*e.g.*, olfaction, nociception) has until recently gone generally unrecognised by the medical community. Accordingly, much remains to be understood on the perceptual-cognitive as well as on the emotional impacts of these proximal sensory cues in infant behaviour and adaptation.

References

1. Lecanuet JP, Schaal B. Foetal sensory competences. *Eur J Obstet Gynecol Reprod Biol* 1996; 68: 1-23.

2. Schaal B, Lecanuet JP, Granier-Deferre C. Sensory and integrative development in the human fetus and perinate: The usefulness of animal models. In: Haug M, Whalen RE, eds. *Animal models of human emotion and cognition*. Washington: American Psychological Association, 1999: 119-42.

3. Lecanuet JP, Fifer WP, Krasnegor NA, Smotherman WP, eds. *Fetal development: A psychobiological perspective*. Orlando, FA: Academic Press, 1995.

4. Hopkins BA, Johnson S, eds. *Prenatal development of postnatal functions*. Mahwah, NJ: Ablex, 2005.

5. Gottlieb, G. Ontogenesis of sensory function in birds and mammals. In: Tobach E, Aronson L, Shaw E, eds, *The biopsychology of development*, New York, NY: Academic Press, 1971: 67-128.

6. Turkewitz G, Kenny PA. The role of developmental limitations of sensory input on sensory/perceptual organization. *Dev Behav Pediatr* 1985; 6: 302-6.

7. Lewkowicz DJ, Lickliter R, eds. *The development of intersensory perception: Comparative perspectives*. Hillsdale, NJ: Erlbaum, 1994.

8. Turkewiz G, Devenny DA, eds. *Developmental time and timing*. Hillsdale, NJ: Erlbaum, 1995.

9. Kenny PA, Turkewitz G. Effect of unusually early visual stimulation on the developing of homing behavior in the rat pup. *Dev Psychobiol* 1986; 19: 57-66.

10. Lickliter R, Banker H. Prenatal components of intersensory development in precocial birds. In: Lewkowicz DJ, Lickliter R, eds. *The development of intersensory perception: comparative perspectives*. Hillsdale, NJ: Erlbaum, 1994: 59-80.

11. Prechtl HFR. The directed Head-turning response and allied movements of the human baby. *Behaviour* 1958; 13: 212-42.

12. Humphrey TM. Functions of the nervous system during prenatal life. In: Stawe U, ed. *Perinatal physiology*. New York, NY: Plenum, 1978: 651-83.

13. Robinson SR, Wong C, Robertson SS, Natanielsz PW, Smotherman WP. Behavioral responses of the chronically instrumented sheep fetus to chemosensory stimuli presented *in utero*. *Behav Neurosci* 1995; 109: 551-62.

14. Schaal B, Coureaud G, Langlois D, Giniès C, Sémon E, Perrier G. Chemical and behavioural characterization of the rabbit mammary pheromone. *Nature* 2003; 424: 68-72.

15. Edelman GM. *Neural darwinism*. New York, NY: Basic Books, 1987.

16. Greenough WT. Experience effects on the developing and the mature brain: Dendritic branching and synaptogenesis. In: Krasnegor NA, Blass EM, Hofer MA, Smotherman WP, eds. *Perinatal development: A psychobiological perspective*. Orlando, FA: Academic Press, 1987: 195-221.

17. Kandel ER, Jessel TM, Sanes JR. Sensory experience and the fine-tuning of synaptic connections. In: Kandel ER, Schwartz JH, Jessel TM, eds. *Principles of neural science*, 4th Edition. New York: McGraw-Hill, 2000: 1116-30.

18. Schneirla. Aspects of stimulation and organization in approach/withdrawal processes underlying vertebrate behavioural development. In: Lehrman DS, Hinde RA, Shaw E, eds. *Advances in the Study of Behavior*. New York, NY: Academic Press, 1965: 1-74.

19. Gottlieb G, Wahlsten D, Lickliter R. The significance of biology for human development: a developmental psychobiological systems view. In: Lerner RM, ed. *Handbook of child Psychology, Vol. 1, Theoretical models of human development*, New York, NY: Wiley, 1998: 233-73.

20. Lickliter R., Bahrick LE. The development of infant intersensory perception: advantages of a comparative convergent-operations approach. *Psychol Bull* 2000; 126: 260-80.

21. Gottlieb G. Experiential canalisation of behavioural development: theory. *Dev Psychol* 1991; 27: 4-13.

22. Smotherman WP, Robinson SR. Tracing developmental trajectories into the prenatal period. In: Lecanuet JP, Fifer WP, Krasnegor NA, Smotherman WP, eds. *Fetal development, A Psychobiological perspective*. Hillsdale, NJ: Erlbaum,1995: 15-32.

23. Schaal B, Orgeur P. Olfaction *in utero*: can the rodent model be generalized? *Quart J Exp Psychol* 1992; 44B: 245-78.

24. DeCasper AJ, Fifer WP. Of human bonding: newborns prefer their mother's voice. *Science* 1980; 208: 1174-76.

25. DeCasper A, Sigafoos AD. The intra uterine heartbeat: a potent reinforcer for newborns. *Infant Behav Dev* 1983; 6: 19-25.

26. DeCasper AJ, Spence M. Prenatal maternal speech influences newborn's perception of speech sounds. *Infant Behav Dev* 1986; 9: 133-50.

27. Schaal B, Marlier L, Soussignan R. Olfactory function in the human fetus: evidence from selective neonatal responsiveness to the odor of amniotic fluid. *Behav Neurosci* 1998; 112: 1-12.

28. Schaal B, Marlier L, Soussignan R. Human foetuses learn odours from their pregnant mother's diet. *Chem Senses* 2000; 25: 729-37.

29. Scafidi F, Field T, Schanberg S, *et al*. Massage stimulates growth in preterm infants: A replication. *Infant Behav Dev* 1990; 13: 167-88.

30. Field TM. Preterm infant massage therapy studies: an American approach. *Semin Neonatol* 2002; 7: 487-94.

31. Blass EM, Ganchrow JR, Steiner JE. Classical conditioning in newborn infants 2-48 hours of age. *Infant Behav Dev* 1984; 7: 483-9.

32. Soussignan R, Schaal B. Emotional processes in human newborns: A functionalist perspective. In: Nadel J, Muir D, eds. *Emotional development: Recent research advances*. Oxford: Oxford University Press, 2004: 127-59.

33. Goren CC, Sarty M, Wu PY. Visual following and pattern discrimination of face-like stimuli by newborn infants. *Pediatrics* 1975; 56: 544-9.

34. Morton J, Johnson MH. CONSPEC and CONLERN: A two-process theory of infant face recognition. *Psychol Rev* 1991; 98: 164-81.

35. Farah MJ, Rabinowitz C, Quinn GE, Liu GT. Early commitment of neural substrates for face recognition. *Cogn Neuropsychol* 2000; 17: 117-23.

36. Schaal B. From amnion to colostrum to milk: odour bridging in early developmental transitions. In: Hopkins BA, Johnson S, eds. *Prenatal development of postnatal functions*. Mahwah, NJ: Ablex, 2005: 52-152.

37. Feijo J. Ut conscientiae noscatue. *Cah Sophrol* 1975; 13: 14-20.

38. Hepper PG. Fetal "soap" addiction. *The Lancet* 1988; 1: 1147-8.

39. Marlier L, Schaal B, Soussignan R. Orientation responses to biological odours in the human newborn. Initial pattern and postnatal plasticity. *CR Acad Sci Paris* 1997; 320: 999-1005.

40. Smotherman WP, Robinson S, La Vallée PA, Hennessy MB. Influences of the early olfactory environment on the survival, behavior and pituitary-adrenal activity of cesarean delivered preterm rat pups. *Dev Psychobiol* 1987; 20: 415-23.

41. Coureaud G, Schaal B, Hudson R, Orgeur P, Coudert P. Transnatal olfactory continuity in the rabbit: Behavioral evidence and short-term consequence of its disruption. *Dev Psychobiol* 2002; 40: 372-90.

42. Marlier L., Schaal B, Soussignan R. Neonatal responsiveness to the odors of amniotic and lacteal fluids: a test of perinatal chemosensory continuity. *Child Dev* 1998; 69: 611-23.

43. Marlier L, Schaal B, Soussignan R. Bottle-fed neonates prefer an odor experienced *in utero* to an odor experienced postnatally in the feeding context. *Dev Psychobiol* 1998; 33: 133-45.

44. Thoman EB, Ingersoll EW. Learning in premature infants. *Dev Psychol* 1993; 29: 692-700.

45. Ferber SG, Kuint J, Weller A, *et al*. Massage therapy by mothers and trained professionals enhances weight gain in preterm infants. *Early Hum Dev* 2002; 67: 37-45.

46. Anderson GC. Kangaroo care of the premature infant. In: Goldson E, ed. *Nurturing the premature infant: developmental interventions in the neonatal intensive care unit*, New York: Oxford University Press, 1999: 131-60.

47. Tessier R, Cristo MB, Velez S, *et al*. Kangaroo mother care: A method for protecting high-risk low-birth-weight and premature infants against developmental delay. *Infant Behav Dev* 2003; 26: 384-97.

48. Mitchell A, Waltman PA. Oral sucrose and pain relief for preterm infants. *Pain Manag Nurs* 2003; 4: 62-9.

49. Schaal B, Hummel T, Soussignan R. Olfaction in the fetal and premature infant: Functional status and clinical implications. *Clin Perinatol* 2004; 31: 261-85.

50. Als H. The preterm infant: A model for the study of fetal brain expectation. In: Lecanuet JP, Fifer WP, Krasnegor NE, Smotherman WP, eds. *Fetal development. A psychobiological Perspective*. Hillsdale, NJ: Lawrence Erlbaum, 1995: 439-71.

51. Kisilewski B, Lecanuet JP. Les connaissances sur l'enfant prématuré bénéficient-elles des recherches sur le fœtus? *Enfance* 1999; 1: 13-26.

52. Hellerud BC, Storm H. Skin conductance and behaviour during sensory stimulation of preterm and term infants. *Early Hum Dev* 2002; 70: 35-46.

53. Rezrazi A, Abdelghani A, Marret S, Mellier D. *Emotional regulation in preterm infants: telethermographic analysis*. 11th European Conference on Developmental Psychology, Milano, Italy, 2003.

54. Fearon I, Kisilewski B, Hains SM, Muir DW, Tranmer J. Swaddling after heel lance: Age specific effects on behavioral recovery in preterm infants. *Dev Behav Pediatr* 1997; 18: 1-11.

Sleep in preterm neonates. Organization, development, deprivation

Véronique Zupan Simunek, Jacques Sizun

General sleep functions

Sleep is a biological process as vital to life as breathing. Its importance for adequate brain function has been frequently proven. The role of paradoxical sleep or rapid eye movement sleep (REM sleep) has been studied extensively. In contrast, less is known about the role of non-REM sleep. In adults, non-REM sleep (or slow wave sleep) is associated with energy restoration and maintenance. REM sleep and non-REM sleep seem homeostatically linked [1].

Sensory input processing

The sleep/waking neural network is modulated by sensory inputs; both sensory deprivation and stimulation may influence this network. REM sleep is involved in processing of sensory information, especially visual inputs [2]. The brain receives a lot of information in wake time that needs to be organized – saved or suppressed – as in a computer system. There are several interactions between the central nervous system (CNS) and sensory inputs that influence normal wake cycling and behaviour [3].

Synaptic efficacy maintenance

REM sleep is involved in dynamic stabilization of infrequently used brain circuits (encoding memories) [2] and is associated with memory consolidation especially during procedural skill learning. According to Kavanau [2] these two functions – dynamic stabilization and sensory information processing – may come into conflict when both occur at a high level and this conflict may have been the selective pressure for sleep's origin.

Hormone, neurotrophic and growth factor secretion

Sleep regulates cortisol and growth hormone [4]. In adults, growth hormone release occurs in the first period of sleep (non-REM sleep). The neurotrophic factor (NGF) has also been associated with sleep [5]. Conversely, several hormones and neuropeptides play a role in sleep regulation [6]. In adults, growth hormone-releasing hormone (GH-RH) induces slow wave sleep and GH secretion, and inhibits cortisol secretion while corticotropin releasing hormone (CRH) has the opposite effect. Galanine, growth hormone releasing peptide and neuropeptide Y also promote sleep. Vasointestinal peptides decelerate the non-REM – REM sleep cycle. Nocturnal sleep onset correlates with melatonin secretion [7].

In infants, the circadian rhythm of cortisol is correlated with the sleep-wake circadian rhythm. Both develop between 8 and 12 weeks of life [8]. Some neuropeptides involved in sleep regulation are also neuroprotective factors. Melatonin has been shown to be highly protective against oxidative stress and excitotoxicity in adult and newborn animals [9, 10]. In human infants, circadian urinary excretion of melatonin has been detected at as early as 4 weeks of life [11]. Low nocturnal melatonin secretion in the first weeks of life correlates with poor psychomotor development [12].

Specific sleep functions during development

Sleep contributes to growth regulation by regulating nutritional supply utilization and growth hormone secretion [13]. It has been hypothesized that sleep is involved in normal development and maturation of the brain [14]. Normal sleep organization is correlated with normal neurological development [15]. Moreover, sleep in early life (specifically REM sleep) may be a promoter of brain development [16].

Sleep organization and maturation

Sleep state organization

In adults, sleep is organized into 5 states: the first 4 states are non-REM sleep, the fifth is REM sleep. Sleep state classification is based on EEG and other recorded physiological parameters such as body movements, eye movements, chin electromyogram (EMG), breathing, and heart rate. The most important parameters for sleep state classification are EEG, regularity of respiration, and presence or absence of rapid eye movements (REM).

In infants under 6 months of age, 3 sleep states have been described [17]:

– Quiet sleep (QS): absence of REM and body movements, presence of regular respiration and tonic chin EMG.

– Active sleep (AS) which approximately corresponds to REM sleep of adults: presence of REM, irregular respiration and body movements, absence of tonic chin EMG.

– Indeterminate sleep (IS): not clearly classifiable as QS or AS. The period of IS at the beginning of sleep and between QS and AS is called transitional sleep.

Sleep states are associated with cyclic variations of the sympathetic-parasympathetic balance: the sympathetic system is dominant during AS whereas the parasympathetic system is dominant during QS [18]. The variability of cerebral blood flow velocity (by doppler measure) is greater in AS than in QS [19]. Well defined states of sleep (AS and QS) are detected at as early as 25 weeks gestational age. Up to term, the predominant state of sleep is AS. The proportion of IS decreases with gestational age: 30% before 34 weeks of postconceptional age, less than 10% of sleep time beyond 35 weeks of postconceptional age [18, 20].

Daily sleeping time in newborns

Daily sleeping time decreases with gestational age [21] or postconceptional age [22]. In preterm infants, it is approximately 18 hours at 32 weeks postconceptional age, and 15 hours at 37 weeks. In full-term infants, sleeping time is around 15 hours on day 1 and 12 hours on day 28.

Sleep-wake organization

Circadian rhythms – the biological clock

The daily sleep-wake rhythm is associated with several physiologic variations (EEG, heart rate, blood pressure, breathing, temperature, etc.) that constitute the circadian rhythms. The circadian clock has been located in the suprachiasmatic nuclei [23]. Circadian rhythms are poorly developed in newborn infants but gradually evolve during the weeks and months after birth. Motor activity, heart rate and blood pressure are not organized in circadian rhythms during the first weeks of life. The sleep-wake rhythm synchronizes with the light-darkness rhythm as at early as one month of life [12]. Conversely, temperature already has a circadian rhythm at birth in full-term infants reflecting activity of the biological clock. Mirmiran and Kok [24] observed a circadian rhythm for temperature at as early as 28 weeks gestational age.

Circadian rhythms in preterm infants

In preterm infants, the maturation of the sleep-wake rhythm after discharge seems independent of environmental factors (light exposure) during the period of hospitalization. It largely depends on postconceptional age [22]. Glotzbach *et al.* [25] studied 17 preterm infants in neonatal intensive care unit (NICU) at 35 weeks postconceptional age: no circadian rhythm was found for activity and heart rate, but very low amplitude circadian rhythms were found for skin and rectal temperature.

As in full-term infants, day-night rhythms become evident at around 8 weeks of postnatal age, and are correlated with the emergence of circadian cortisol secretion [26].

Ultradian rhythm

In adults, there is a periodicity in CNS activity throughout the day which corresponds with the rest-activity cycle. A periodicity of approximately 90 min is measurable by EEG. Ultradian rhythms of CNS activity (eye movements) have been recorded in the foetus at as early as 20 weeks gestation [27]. Wakayama et al. [27] recorded ultradian rhythms of EEG in newborn infants of 25 to 42 weeks gestation: most rhythm periods were shorter than 30 min.

Ultradian rhythms of activity are correlated with environmental factors, especially with feeding. In the NICU, ultradian rhythms of preterm infants for temperature, activity and heart rate are correlated with feedings and related interventions [25].

Control of the sleep organization

In adults, REM sleep, generated within the brain stem, particularly within the pons, is characterized by induction of intense tonic and phasic central activation and inhibition of sensory input and motor output [28]. Cholinergic, GABAergic and serotoninergic neurons in the medial medullary reticular formation contribute to regulation of sleep-wake regulation and control of muscle tone during REM sleep [29]. In infants with a normal brain, developmental changes of sleep organization depend only on postconceptional age; they seem independent of environmental factors. Sleep organization reflects the maturation of CNS, in particular of the brain-stem [30].

Effects of environment on the sleep

Sleep deprivation

Animal studies

Animal studies suggest that sleep deprivation has an unfavourable short and long term impact.

Recent researches in animal models have demonstrated changes in respiratory behaviour, brain neurochemistry and brain receptor density induced by pharmacological suppression of AS sleep in the neonatal period [31, 32]. Rat pups deprived of REM sleep present at adult age with behavioural and attention disorders and reduced cerebral cortical size [33]. These changes are not modified by subsequent environmental enrichment [34, 35].

Moderate sleep deprivation in humans

In healthy adults, moderate sleep deprivation is associated with significant cognitive and motor impairments. Moreover, sleep deprivation affects the individual's mood [36]. In normal full-term newborns, moderate deprivation of sleep does not alter the sleep organization but increases the number of obstructive respiratory events during AS [37].

Sleep and hospitalization in intensive care unit (ICU)

In adult intensive care units (ICU), sleep deprivation has been reported by patients, families and staff to be one of the major stress factors [38]. In fact, severe sleep fragmentation has been observed in all types of adult ICUs, with a high frequency of arousals and awakenings [39] and daytime sleepiness [40]. In ICU hospitalized adults, sleep deprivation is associated with impairment of normal melatonin secretion [41]. The role of sleep disruption in the genesis of ICU psychosis is currently being discussed [42]. The environmental aetiologies of sleep disruption in the ICU are multifactorial [40], but noise appears as the main causative factor [43]. Many of the ICU noises seem amenable to the staff's behavioural changes [44]. Sleep deprivation was also reported in paediatric ICUs with an evident link to noise, light and caregiver activity [45].

There is an evident lack of information on the quality of babies' sleep in newborn intensive care units (NICU). Consequences of sleep suppression in full-term and preterm neonates on further neurobehavioural outcome are unknown. Non-circadian care does not alter the development of circadian rhythm in preterm infants, but interventions and abnormal environments associated with NICU exposure may induce important biological effects, not studied up to now [46].

Effects of environmental factors on sleep organization in term and preterm infants

The effects of deprivation of maternal environment after premature birth are not well known.

Most environmental factors can interfere with AS/QS ratio and/or daily time of sleep:

– Temperature: exposure to cool environments increases AS duration [47].

– Posture: prone and side-lying nested are comfortable positions which are associated with less stressful behaviour and longer periods of light sleep in preterm infants [48]. In full-term infants, prone position is associated with longer QS but also with more adverse respiratory events (apnoea, failure to arousal). This association has not been found in preterm infants.

– Type of feeding: formulas with medium chain triglycerides increase body temperature and total sleep time in premature infants and increase the proportion of AS [49].

Effects of drugs

Sedative and analgesic drugs alter EEG ground activity inducing low voltage and discontinuity. The long term effects of such drugs routinely administered in NICU infants are unknown. Infants of drug or alcohol-dependent mothers exhibit behaviour and sleep disorders beyond the phase of withdrawal. Altered sleep with abnormal arousal responses has been described in infants exposed to cigarette smoke [50]. Corticosteroids, which were sometimes administered for a long period in infants with bronchopulmonary dysplasia, may also disturb sleep organization.

Effects of developmental care in preterm newborn infants

NICU caregivers are aware that babies experience pain, discomfort and sleep disturbance. Individualized developmental care has been proposed in order to improve the quality of life of preterm babies, particularly by respecting rest and sleep time. The Newborn Individualized Developmental Care and Assessment Program (NIDCAP) showed short term benefits on ventilation and feeding [51], but failed to demonstrate substantial improvement of sleep time in preterm infants [52]. In a cross-over trial with sleep duration as main outcome, Bertelle *et al.* demonstrated an increase in total and quiet sleep with developmental care [53].

Effects of neurological and non-neurological diseases on sleep development

Neurological diseases

Severe neurological diseases (cystic periventricular leukomalacia, hypoxic-ischemic encephalopathy, etc.) are clearly associated with sleep EEG abnormalities, particularly in QS. Some of these neurologically impaired infants also develop sleep disorders.

Respiratory diseases

Infants with upper airway obstruction have a significantly smaller proportion of AS sleeping time [54]. Sleep is altered in infants with chronic hypoxemia caused by bronchopulmonary dysplasia. These infants also show growth failure.

Growth retardation

Newborns with intrauterine growth retardation (IUGR) frequently exhibit a characteristic behaviour pattern of excitability and sleepiness. Some of these IUGR babies often have altered sleep organization [55] and can develop delayed EEG maturation which is correlated with poor cognitive development [56]. Postnatal malnutrition may also alter neurological development. Interestingly, attention deficit/hyperactivity disorder (ADHD), which is frequent in children born preterm or small for gestational age, is associated with sleep disturbances [57].

Conclusion

Animal studies are consistent with the hypothesis that sleep, and specifically REM sleep, is an important factor for normal brain development. Sleep organization and maturation depend on both endogenous and environmental factors. Several animal studies have demonstrated the long term impact of early sleep deprivation on subsequent neurodevelopment. Human studies have reported adverse sleep deprivation outcomes in adult hospitalized in ICU. Some observations may be found in the NICU inasmuch as recognition of babies' sleep states appears clinically available for staff, even for preterm infants. The gap between research and evidence-based practice for effective sleep protection in hospitalized neonates remains wide, as previously demonstrated for neonatal pain control. A circadian environmental approach in NICU is recommended with implementation of nursing care which is associated with babies' sleep-based schedule.

Acknowledgements

The authors thank Dr. Dominique Samson-Dollfuss for helpful discussions and Dr. Annette Scheid for their linguistic help.

References

1. Benington JH, Heller HC. Does the function of REM sleep concern non-REM sleep or waking? *Prog Neurobiol* 1994; 44: 433-49.

2. Kavanau JL. Memory, sleep and the evolution of mechanisms of synaptic efficacy maintenance. *Neuroscience* 1997; 79: 7-44.

3. Velluti RA. Interactions between sleep and sensory physiology. *J Sleep Res* 1997; 6: 61-77.

4. Van Cauter E, Leproult R, Plat L. Age-related changes in slow wave sleep and REM sleep and relationship with growth hormone and cortisol levels in healthy men. *JAMA* 2000; 284: 861-8.

5. Sei H, Saitoh D, Yamamoto K, Morita K, Morita Y. Differential effect of short-term REM sleep deprivation on NGF and BDNF protein levels in the rat brain. *Brain Res* 2000; 22: 387-90.

6. Steiger A, Holsboer F. Neuropeptides and human sleep. *Sleep* 1997; 20: 1038-52.

7. Lewy J, Ahmed S, Latham Jackson J, Sack R. Melatonin shifts human circadian rhythms according to phase curve. *Chronobiol Int* 1992; 9: 380-92.

8. Santiago LB, Jorge SM, Moreira AC. Longitudinal evaluation of the development of salivary cortisol circadian rhythm in infancy. *Clin Endocrinol* 1996; 44: 157-61.

9. Chung SY, Han SH. Melatonin attenuates kainic acid-induced hippocampal neurodegeneration and oxidative stress through microglial inhibition. *J Pineal Res* 2003; 34: 95-102.

10. Husson I, Mesples B, Bac P, Vamecq J, Evrard P, Gressens P. Melatoninergic neuroprotection of the murine periventricular white matter against neonatal excitotoxic challenge. *Ann Neurol* 2002; 51: 82-92.

11. Ardura J, Gutierrez R, Andres J, Agapito T. Emergence and evolution of the circadian rhythm of melatonin in children. *Horm Res* 2003; 59: 66-72.

12. Tauman R, Zisapel N, Laudon M, Nehama H, Sivan Y. Melatonin production in infants. *Pediatr Neurol* 2002; 26: 379-82.

13. Salzarulo P, Fagioli I. Sleep for development or development for waking? Some speculations from human perspective. *Behav Brain Res* 1995; 69: 23-7.

14. Mirmiran M. The function of fetal/neonatal rapid eye movement sleep. *Behav Brain Res* 1995; 69: 13-22.

15. Whitney MP, Thoman EB. Early sleep patters of premature infants are differentially related to later developmental disabilities. *J Dev Behav Pediatr* 1993; 14: 71-80.

16. Mirmiran M, Van Someren E. Normal and abnormal REM sleep regulation: The importance of REM sleep for brain maturation. *J Sleep Res* 1993; 2: 188-92.

17. Curzi-Dascalova L, Challamel MJ. Neurophysiological basis of sleep development. In: Loughlin GM, Carroll JL, Marcus CL, eds. *Sleep and breathing in children. A developmental approach*. New York: Marcel Dekker, 2000: 3-37.

18. Curzi-Dascalova L, Figueroa JM, Eiselt M, Christova E, Virassamy A, d'Allest AM, Guimaraes H, Gaultier C, Dehan M. Sleep state organization in premature infants of less than 35 weeks' gestational age. *Pediatr Res* 1993; 34: 624-8.

19. Rehan VK, Fajardo CA, Haider AZ, et al. Influence of sleep state and respiratory pattern on cyclical fluctuations of cerebral blood flow velocity in healthy preterm infants. *Biol Neonate* 1996; 69: 357-67.

20. Curzi-Dascalova L, Peirano P, Morel-Kahn F. Development of sleep states in normal premature and full-term newborns. *Dev Psychobiol* 1988; 21: 431-44.

21. Ardura J, Andrés J, Aldana J, Revilla MA. Development of sleep-wakefulness rhythm in premature babies. *Acta Paediatr* 1995; 84: 484-9.

22. Shimada M, Segawa M, Higurashi M, Akamatsu H. Development of the sleep and wakefulness rhythm in preterm infants discharged from a neonatal care unit. *Pediatr Res* 1993; 33: 159-63.

23. Rivkees SA. Developing circadian rhythmicity in infants. *Pediatrics* 2003; 112: 373-81.

24. Mirmiran M, Kok, JH. Circadian rhythms in early human development. *Early Hum Dev* 1991; 26: 121-8.

25. Glotzbach SF, Edgar DM, Ariagno RL. Biological rhythmicity in preterm infants prior to discharge from neonatal intensive care. *Pediatrics* 1995; 95: 231-7.

26. Antonini SR, Jorge SM, Moreira AC. The emergence of salivary cortisol circadian rhythm and its relationship to sleep activity in preterm infants. *Clin Endocrinol* 2000; 52: 423-6.

27. Wakayama K, Ogawa T, Goto K, Sonoda H. Developement of ultradian rhythm of EEG activities in premature babies. *Early Hum Dev* 1993; 32: 11-30.

28. Jones BE. Paradoxical sleep and its chemical/structural substrates in the brain. *Neuroscience* 1991; 40: 637-56.

29. Holmes CJ, Jones BE. Importance of cholinergic, GABAergic, serotoninergic and other neurons in the medial medullary reticular formation for sleep-wake states studied by excitotoxic lesions in the cat. *Neuroscience* 1994; 62: 1179-200.

30. Kohyama J, Iwakawa Y. Developmental changes in phasic sleep parameters as reflections of brain-stem maturation: polysomnoraphical examinations of infants, including premature neonates. *Electroencephalogr Clin Neurophysiol* 1990; 76: 325-30.

31. Thomas AJ, Erokwu BO, Yamamoto BK, Ernsberger P, Bishara O, Strohl KP. Alterations in respiratory behavior, brain neurochemistry and receptor density induced by pharmacologic suppression of sleep in the neonatal period. *Dev Brain Res* 2000; 120: 181-9.

32. Létourneau P, Niyonsenga T, Carrier E, Praud E, Praud JP. Influence of 24-Hour sleep deprivation on respiration in Lambs. *Pediatr Res* 2002; 52: 697-705.

33. Mirmiran M. The importance of fetal/neonatal REM sleep. *Eur J Obstet Gynecol Reprod Biol* 1986; 21: 283-91.

34. Mirmiran M, Scholtens J, van de Poll NE, Uylings HB, van der Gugten J, Boer GJ. Effects of experimental suppression of active (REM) sleep during early development upon adult brain and behavior in the rat. *Brain Res* 1983; 283: 277-86.

35. Mirmiran M, Uylings HB, Corner MA. Pharmacological suppression of REM sleep prior to weaning counteracts the effectiveness of subsequent environmental enrichment on cortical growth in rats. *Brain Res* 1983; 283: 102-5.

36. Pilcher JJ, Huffcutt AI. Effects of sleep deprivation on performance: a meta-analysis. *Sleep* 1996; 19: 318-26.

37. Canet E, Gaultier C, d'Allest AM, Dehan M. Effects of sleep deprivation on respiratory events during sleep in healthy infants. *J Appl Physiol* 1989; 66: 1158-63.

38. Novaes MA, Knobel E, Bork AM, Pavao OF, Nogueira-Martins LA, Ferraz MB. Stressors in ICU: perception of the patient, relatives and health care team. *Intensive Care Med* 1999; 25: 1421-6.

39. Cooper AB, Thornley KS, Young GB, Slutsky AS, Stewart TE, Hanly PJ. Sleep in critically ill patients requiring mechanical ventilation. *Chest* 2000; 117: 809-18.

40. Freedman NS, Kotzer N, Schwab RJ. Patient perception of sleep quality and etiology of sleep disruption in the intensive care unit. *Am J Respir Crit Care Med* 1999; 159: 1155-62.

41. Shilo L, Dagan Y, Smorjik Y, et al. Patients in the intensive care unit suffer from severe lack of sleep associated with loss of normal melatonin secretion pattern. *Am J Med Sci* 1999; 317: 278-81.

42. McGuire BE, Basten CJ, Ryan CJ, Gallagher J. Intensive care unit syndrome: a dangerous misnomer. *Arch Intern Med* 2000; 160: 906-9.

43. Aaron JN, Carlisle CC, Carskadon MA, Meyer TJ, Hill NS, Millman RP. Environmental noise as a cause of sleep disruption in an intermediate respiratory care unit. *Sleep* 1996; 19: 707-10.

44. Kahn DM, Cook TE, Carlisle CC, Nelson DL, Kramer NR, Millman RP. Identification and modification of environmental noise in an ICU setting. *Chest* 1998; 114: 535-40.

45. Cureton-Lane RA, Fontaine DK. Sleep in the pediatric ICU: an empirical investigation. *Am J Crit Care* 1997; 6: 56-63.

46. Mirmiran M, Ariagno RL. Influence of light in the NICU on the development of circadian rhythms in preterm infants. *Semin Perinatol* 2000; 24: 247-57.

47. Bach V, Bouferrache B, Kremp O, Maingourd Y, Libert JP. Regulation of sleep and body temperature in response to exposure to cool and warm environment in neonates. *Pediatrics* 1994; 93: 789-96.

48. Grenier IR, Bigsby R, Vergara ER, Lester BM. Comparison of motor self-regulatory and stress behaviors of preterm infants across body positions. *Am J Occup Ther* 2003; 57: 289-97.

49. Telliez F, Bach V, Dewasmes G, Leke A, Libert JP. Effects of medium- and long-chain triglycerides on sleep and thermoregulatory processes in neonates. *J Sleep Res* 1998; 7: 31-9.

50. Chang AB, Wilson SJ, Masters IB, et al. Altered arousal response in infants exposed to cigarette smoke. *Arch Dis Child* 2003; 88: 30-3.

51. Als H, Lawhon G, Duffy FH, McAnulty GB, Gibes-Grossman R, Blickman JG. Individualized developmental care for the very low-birth-weight preterm infant. Medical and neurofunctional effects. *JAMA* 1994; 272: 853-8.

52. Westrup B, Hellstrom-Westas L, Stjernqvist K, Lagercrantz H. No indications of increased quiet sleep in infants receiving care based on the newborn individualized developmental care and assessment program (NIDCAP). *Acta Paediatr* 2002; 91: 318-22.

53. Bertelle V, Mabin D, Adrien J, Sizun J. Sleep of preterm neonates under developmental care or regular environmental conditions. *Early Hum Dev* 2005; 81: 595-600.

54. McNamara F, Sullivan CE. Sleep-disordered breathing and its effects on sleep in infants. *Sleep* 1996; 19: 4-12.

55. Arduini D, Rizzo G, Caforio L, Boccolini MR, Romanini C, Mancuso S. Behavioural state transitions in healthy and growth retarded fetuses. *Early Hum Dev* 1989. 19: 155-65.

56. Okumura A, Hayakawa F, Kato T, et al. Developmental outcome and types of chronic-stage EEG abnormalities in preterm infants. *Dev Med Child Neurol* 2002; 44: 729-34.

57. O'Brien LM, Ivanenko A, Crabtree VM, et al. Sleep disturbances in children with attention deficit hyperactivity disorder. *Pediatr Res* 2003; 54: 237-43.

Neonatal development: Effects of light

Dominique Haumont, Valérie Hansen

Preterm infants are at high risk for adverse neurodevelopmental and sensory outcome. A 15-25% incidence of disability has been reported in follow-up studies of very-low-birth-weight infants (VLBWI, < 1500 g) and up to 50% in extremely-low-birth-weight infants (ELBWI, < 1000 g) [1-5]. The developing visual system can be impacted in many ways since it is the last of the sensory systems to fully develop. Cortical vision impairment and retinopathy are possible consequences of preterm birth. More subtle vision impairments are also related to prematurity *per se*. The factors associated with adverse outcome are multiple and subject to continuous debate. The aim of the present article is to review the influence of light on neonatal development.

The amount of light reaching the neonatal eye

Physical and physiological factors determine the amount of light reaching the infant's eye in the neonatal unit. Illumination levels of neonatal intensive care units (NICU) are often high and continuous. The impact of this light environment may be influenced by particular aspects of the immature infant's development. In understanding the impact of light on the preterm neonatal eye, specific anatomical and physiological characteristics merit discussion. Eyelid opening is related to the illumination of the NICU and the infant's developmental stage. At 28 weeks gestation, babies monitored for 24 continuous hours, have their eyes shut during 93% of the time observed. At 26 weeks gestation, their eyes were open only during 55% of the observation time. Neonates exposed to continuous illumination closed their eyes more than babies under a cycled light regimen [6]. Retinal irradiance is also dependant on pupil size. The pupillary light reflex appears only after 30 weeks of gestation and mydriasis is physiological until 32 weeks. The pupillary diameter decreases from ± 4.7 mm at 26 weeks to ± 3.3 mm at 29-30 weeks [7].

The amount of light reaching the retina depends on the eyelids and inner ocular tissues like the cornea, aqueous and the crystalline lens. They filter out most radiation below 400 nm [8]. The peak transmission in preterm infants is at the red end of the spectrum (700 nm) and is twice as high when compared to the adult eye [9]. Based on these studies, retinal irradiance has been estimated to decrease from 530 µW/cm² at 24 weeks to 250 µW/cm² at 31 weeks gestation. Therefore, when studying the amount of light reaching the neonatal eye, the characteristics of the preterm eye have to be considered.

Effects of light on the retina and oxydative stress

Visual maturation at term requires adequate stimulation. Binocular and monocular deprivation in early infancy has been demonstrated to induce amblyopia [10]. Light also acts as a stimulus for the production of free radicals in retinal membrane lipids. It has been suggested that the immature antioxidant status of the preterm infant might play a role in their susceptibility to retinal damage. Oxidative stress injury is now considered as being a major contributor to several perinatal diseases like brain damage, retinopathy of prematurity, bronchopulmonary dysplasia and enterocolitis [11]. Factors responsible for oxidative stress in preterm infants include oxygen therapy, immature antioxidant defences, administration of long chain poly-unsaturated fatty acids, infections and undernutrition. Recently the role of phototherapy and light has been underlined as a potential inducer of lipid hydroperoxides in babies receiving parenteral nutrition with lipids and even in babies receiving enteral formula [12, 13]. Lipid infusion lines themselves must be protected from phototherapy light sources in clinical practice.

Light and retinopathy of prematurity (ROP)

With the increasing survival of ELBWI the absolute numbers of infants with ROP remains high. The Vermont Oxford Network 1998 reported an incidence of 80% in infants below a birth weight of 700 grams. Oxygen, free radicals, vascular factors and mainly immaturity are factors contributing to the development of the disease. Exposure to light has been suggested as a cause of ROP since 1943 [14]. Several studies were undertaken but a recent large prospective randomized multicenter study could not demonstrate any direct effect of light on retinopathy [15]. However, this doesn't mean that the debate is closed. In the study cited, the infants were protected from light by wearing goggles, but no attention was paid to light reduction in the unit or to cycled lighting. It has been demonstrated that reducing ambient light and noise has indirect effects on staff behaviour leading to less handling and less stressful procedures for babies in the NICU [16, 17]. Thus, the confounding effects of fewer environmental interruptions and interventions associated with reduced lighting have yet to be clarified.

Light and ophthalmic sequelae of prematurity *per se*

Preterm infants often show visual impairment even without ROP, due to neurological damage and premature birth. Ophthalmic sequelae of preterm birth include reduced visual acuity, colour vision, and contrast sensitivity. Strabismus and myopia are also common consequences of preterm birth. Etiological factors are not well understood, but environmental factors like ambient light or corneal temperature have been implicated. In a prospective follow-up study at 5 years of age, deficits in visuospatial and sensorimotor function were detected and attributed to damage of the brain stem and thalamic structures regulating sensory input under the control of higher cortical structures [18]. Recent studies on ophthalmic and cerebral blood flow velocities have demonstrated increases of blood flow induced by increasing ambient light or by phototherapy [19, 20]. Regional hemodynamic responses to light measured by near-infrared spectroscopy showed an increased cerebral blood flow in the visual cortex [21]. Future research is needed to establish the role of these hemodynamic responses to light in the developmental process of preterm infants.

Effect of light on the circadian rhythms

Human physiology shows a circadian rhythmicity endogenously driven over a 24 hour period. The biological clock is located in the hypothalamic suprachiasmatic nuclei (SCN) at the base of the third ventricle. Input pathways entrained by light are relayed to the SCN which express output signals. These include temperature, cortisol, melatonin, sleep-wake-cycle, behaviour and cardiovascular function [22]. *In utero* the fetus has a biological clock that responds to maternal entraining signals. If the baby is born preterm he will be deprived of this maternally regulated circadian rhythm and will be submitted to an often chaotic and bright NICU environment. Studies in a premature non-human primate model have shown significant responsiveness of the biological clock to bright light in at a gestational age equivalent to 24 weeks in humans. Indeed, the biological clock, responded to light by increasing SCN metabolic activity and gene expression [23].

In preterm infants, several studies have shown that they have ultradian rhythms (period lengths much less than 24 hours). It is likely that these ultradian rhythms are driven by care giving and mask or disrupt the appearance of circadian rhythms [24]. Attention is now directed towards the impact of environmental factors on the infant's development. The Newborn Individualised Developmental Care and Assessment Program (NIDCAP) addresses in a very physiological way the complexity of the impact of the environment on preterm infant behaviour and supports lowering lighting levels in the NICU [25]. Even more importantly, NIDCAP recommends individual assessment and adaptation of the impact of environmental factors among which light has an important role.

Lighting policies in the NICU are still under investigation. The subject has been considered important by the American Academy of Pediatrics and The American College of Obstetricians and Gynaecologists [26]. The recent Guidelines for Perinatal Care recommend lighting levels of 10 to 600 lux (1080 lux for procedures) and a regular day-night cycle in the NICU. However, eduction of light levels does not necessarily meet staff needs. Separate rooms with different lighting should be designed for specific tasks. Bright light is required for preparation of drugs, staff rounds or relaxing rooms for staff and parents.

Conclusions

The effect of light on development in the perinatal period has been fairly extensively investigated. There is substantial evidence in animal, basic and clinical research of the impact of light on physiological processes. A direct relationship between light and clinical outcome variables is difficult to establish because of the multifactorial aspects of what happens to a preterm infant in the NICU. Nevertheless, there is enough background research to consider the influence of light in future research in terms of direct and indirect effects. The worrying neurobehavioral outcomes of ELBW infants should stimulate all our efforts to enhance their future quality of life. Extremely common habits like switching lights on and off, covering the incubators or not or starting the most current treatment like phototherapy should be regarded with knowledge of their potential impact on the developing brain. More research is needed to enhance our insight in this field.

References

1. Escobar GJ, Littenberg B, Petitti DB. Outcome among surviving very low birth weight infants: a meta-analysis. *Arch Dis Child* 1991; 66: 204-11.

2. Cooke RW. Factors affecting survival and outcome at 3 years in extremely preterm infants. *Arch Dis Child* 1994; 71: F28-31.

3. Bylund B, Cervin T, Finnstrom O, et al. Morbidity and neurological function of very low birth weight infants from the newborn period to 4 years of age. A prospective study from the south-east region of Sweden. *Acta Paediatr* 1998; 87: 758-63.

4. Finnstrom O, Otterblad Olausson P, Sedin G, et al. Neurosensory outcome and growth at three years in extremely low birth weight infants: follow-up results from the Swedish national prospective study. *Acta Paediatr* 1998; 87: 1055-60.

5. Vohr BR, Wright LL, Dusick AM, et al. Neurodevelopmental and functional outcomes of extremely low birth weight infants in the National Institute of Child Health and Human Development Neonatal Research Network, 1993-1994. *Pediatrics* 2000; 105: 1216-26.

6. Robinson J, Moseley MJ, Thompson JR, Fielder AR. Eyelid opening in preterm neonates. *Arch Dis Child* 1989; 64: 943-8.

7. Isenberg SJ, Molarte A, Vazquez M. The fixed and dilated pupils of premature neonates. *Am J Ophthalmol* 1990; 110: 168-71.

8. Ludwigh WE, McCarthy EF. Absorption of visible light by the refractive components of the human eye. *Arch Ophthalmol* 1938; 20: 37-51.

9. Robinson J, Bayliss SC, Fielder AR. Transmission of light across the adult and neonatal eyelid *in vivo*. *Vision Res* 1991; 31: 35-8.

10. Crawford M.L. The visual deprivation syndrome. *Ophthalmology* 1978; 85: 465-77.

11. Saugstad OD. Is oxygen more toxic than currently believed? *Pediatrics* 2001; 108: 1203-5.

12. Neuzil L, Darlow BA, Inder TE, Sluis KB, Winterbourn CC, Stocker R. Oxidation of parenteral lipid emulsion by ambient and phototherapy lights potential toxicity of routine parenteral feeding. *J Pediatr* 1995; 126: 785-90.

13. Van Zoeren Grobben D, Moison RM, Ester WM, Berger HM. Lipid peroxidation in human milk and infant formula: effect of storage, tube feeding and exposure to phototherapy. *Acta Paediatr* 1993; 82: 645-9.

14. Terry TL. Fibroplastic overgrowth of persistent tunica vasculosa lentis in premature infants. II. Report of cases – clinical aspects. *Arch Ophtalm* 1943; 29: 36-53.

15. Reynolds JD, Hardy RJ, Kennedy KA, Spencer R, van Heuven WA, Fielder AR. Lack of efficacy of light reduction in preventing retinopathy of prematurity. *N Engl J Med* 1998; 338: 1572-6.

16. Fielder AR, Moseley MJ. Environmental light and the preterm infant. *Semin Perinatol* 2000; 24: 291-8.

17. Mann NP, Haddow R, Stokes L, Goodley S, Rutter N. Effect of night and day on preterm infants in a newborn nursery randomised trial. *Br Med J* 1986; 293: 1265-7.

18. Luoma L, Herrgard E, Martikainen A. Neuropsychological analysis of the visuomotor problems in children born preterm at ≤ 32 weeks of gestation: a 5-year prospective follow-up. *Dev Med Child Neurol* 1998; 40: 21-30.

19. Baerts W, Valentin RAC, Sauer PJJ. Ophthalmic and cerebral blood flow velocities in preterm infants: influence of ambient lighting conditions. *J Clin Ultrasound* 1992; 20: 43-8.

20. Benders MJNL, Van Bel F, Van de Bor M. The effect of phototherapy on cerebral blood flow velocity in preterm infants. *Acta Paediatr* 1998; 87: 786-91.

21. Meek JH, Firbank M, Elwell CE, Atkinson J, Braddick O, Wyatt JS. Regional hemodynamic responses to visual stimulation in awake infants. *Pediatr Res* 1998; 43: 840-3.

22. Moore-Ede MC, Czeisler CA, Richardson GS. Circadian timekeeping in health and disease. Part I. Basic properties of circadian pacemakers. *N Engl J Med* 1983; 309: 469-76.

23. Hao H, Rivkees SA. The biological clock of very premature primate infants is responsive to light. *Neurobiology* 1999; 96: 2426-29.

24. Rivkees SA, Hao H. Developing circadian rhythmicity. *Semin Perinatol* 2000; 24: 232-42.

25. Als H, Lawhon G, Duffy FH, McAnulty GB, Gibes-Grossman R, Blickman JG. Individualized developmental care for the very low-birth-weight preterm infant. Medical and neurofunctional effects. *JAMA* 1994; 272: 835-88.

26. American Academy of Pediatrics and The American College of Obstetricians and Gynecologists. *Guidelines for Perinatal Care*. 4th ed. Elk Grove Village, IL and Washington, DC: American Academy of Pediatrics and The American College of Obstetricians and Gynecologists, 1997.

Effects of positioning and handling on preterm infants in the neonatal intensive care unit

Karl Bauer

The neonatal intensive care unit (NICU) environment of the preterm infant is very different from the intrauterine environment of the foetus. Among the many differences are gravity and handling by parents, medical, and nursing staff. This chapter will review the effects of positioning and of non-painful handling on cardiovascular and respiratory function, on sleep state, arousal, and on neurodevelopment with emphasis on studies whose results have influenced today's standard practices in the NICU.

Positioning

In preterm infants the effects of head-up *versus* head-down tilts and of prone *versus* supine sleep position have been studied. Tilts are acute changes of position within a few minutes, whereas in studies comparing prone or supine sleep positions the respective positions were assigned for periods of 3-6 hours.

Head up *versus* head down tilts

The short term effects of acute head-up or head-down tilts have been studied to investigate baroreceptor control of heart rate and blood pressure in preterm infants. The acute positional change by a head-up tilt results in a transient small drop of blood pressure which is compensated by an increase in heart rate, whereas a head down tilt results in a decrease in heart rate. This reflex was shown to be already well-developed in term infants on day 1 of life and resulted in an increase of heart rate by 1 bpm for each 10° of head-up tilt. This increase was accompanied by a decrease in respiratory rate of 1 breath per minute for each 10° tilt [1]. In preterm infants of 28-32 weeks, this reflex could not be consistently demonstrated, but with increasing postnatal age the reflex response became more marked [2]. Acute head-up and head-down tilts have also been utilised to study the autoregulation of cerebral perfusion in neonates between 24-41 weeks gestation. Sporadic autoregulatory responses were found even in very immature infants. The reliability of making an active autoregulatory response to tilting increased with gestational age [3]. A 30° head up position similar to that during skin-to-skin care was well tolerated by preterm infants [4].

Prone *versus* supine sleeping position

Prone *versus* supine sleeping positions of preterm infants have been studied extensively. The effects which were examined can be grouped in 4 broad categories: respiration, cardiac activity, sleep and arousal, and reduction of morbidity *(table I)*. Usually a cross-over design was used, and the majority of studies included a small sample size. The respective position was assigned for a period of only several hours. The results of these studies are only valid for preterm infants cared for in the environment of the NICU.

Table I. Effects of the prone compared to the supine position in preterm infants.

Effects of prone position on respiration
- Increased tidal volume [5]
- Increased respiratory rate [6]
- Reduced the work of breathing [7]
- Increased transcutaneous oxygen tension [6, 9]

Effects of prone position on cardiovascular activity
- Higher heart rate and lower heart rate variability [12]

Effects of prone position on sleep and arousal
- Less time spent awake and decrease in energy expenditure [14]
- More time spent in quiet sleep [13]
- Less awakenings from sleep [15]

Effects of prone position on morbidity
- Reduced number of apnoeas [11, 16]
- Reduction in the severity of gastro-oesophageal reflux [17]
- Less hypoxic episodes in preterm infants with chronic lung disease [10]

Effects on respiration

The prone position increased tidal volume [5], increased respiratory rate [6] and reduced the work of breathing [7]. The improved respiration resulted in better oxygenation with an increase in arterial pO_2 in the prone compared to the supine position [8, 9]. Moreover, preterm infants lying prone had more reserve for increasing their ventilation in response to hypercapnia [6]. The improvement in respiration by using the prone position was found in ventilated preterm infants [5], in preterm infants with chronic lung disease [10], in preterm infants with apnoea [11], and in preterm infants free of clinically significant respiratory disease shortly before discharge [6]. Mechanisms proposed to explain these effects of the prone position were improved ventilation-perfusion matching, decreased asynchronous chest wall movements, and facilitation of the work of breathing. Changes in the work of breathing were thought to be due to the abdominal contents falling away from the posterior portion of the diaphragm, therefore this area of greatest diaphragmatic excursions moves more freely and with less muscular work.

Effects on cardiac activity

The higher heart rate and lower heart rate variability found in preterm infants lying prone suggest an increased sympathetic dominance in this position [12].

Effects on sleep and arousal

Preterm infants lying prone spent less time awake [13, 14] and had fewer awakenings [15]. Less awake activity decreased energy expenditure in the prone compared to the supine sleeping position [14].

Reduction of morbidity

While lying prone, preterm infants had less apnoea [11, 16] and preterm infants with chronic lung disease had fewer hypoxic episodes [10]. Prone positioning also reduced the severity of gastro-oesophageal reflux [17].

Effects of non-painful handling during medical and nursing care procedures

Non-painful handling of preterm infants occurs during medical and nursing care, but also during social interaction with caregivers and parents. This chapter focusses on non-painful handling during medical and nursing care procedures. Handling associated with pain and handling in the context of neurodevelopmental stimulation for preterm infants are reviewed in other chapters of this book.

There are many studies of short term changes in cardiopulmonary parameters or behavioural state caused by non-painful handling demonstrating the immature and fragile regulatory mechanisms of preterm infants. One type of handling occurs during interventions necessary for survival and clinical well-being of preterm infants. Among those, endotracheal suctioning is a relatively stressful intervention that results in blood pressure changes [18], a decrease in oxygen saturation and cerebral oxygenation [19], an increase in adrenaline and noradrenaline levels [20], and an increase in oxygen consumption [21]. One study [22] which examined the incidence of an acute drop in transcutaneously measured paO_2 provides a rough grading of the stressfulness of different routine care procedure *(table II)*. Other physiological effects observed during routine nursing care were a decrease in rectal temperature [23], increases in skin blood flow [24], and an estimated 2 to 12% increase in daily oxygen consumption caused by unrest due to medical care procedures [21].

Table II. Proportions of infants exhibiting an acute decrease in T_cPO_2 following different routine care procedures (from Danford et al. 1983 [22]).

	Infants with acute decrease in transcutaneous oxygen tension (t_cpO_2) (%)
Chest X-ray	100
Changing the t_cO_2 electrode	60
Physiotherapy	55
Weighing	50
Taking vital signs	50
Tube feeding	50
Diaper change	29

Procedures regarded at first glance as "benign" can also destabilize preterm infants. Taking vital signs resulted in an acute fall in transcutaneously measured pO_2 in 50% of infants studied [22]. Preterm infants who were handled by positioning before a routine heel stick exhibited significantly greater physiologic responses and behavioural arousal to the heelstick compared with infants who had not been handled [25]. Fluctuations in cerebral oxygenation were observed when incubator doors were opened or conversations were held near the incubator [26]. Performing a neurobehavioural assessment involving reflex testing and repositioning (Brazelton Neonatal Assessment Scale) resulted in elevated cortisol levels [27]. Even procedures intended to "protect" the infants can in fact destabilize them. For example, local analgesia before a lumbar puncture did not reduce the physiological instability of the preterm infant. Instead, the additional handling associated with providing the local analgesia was more destabilizing than the short acute pain [28].

Conclusion

The studies reviewed here have shaped the current standard concepts of positioning and handling in the neonatal intensive care unit. Positioning (head-up, prone versus supine) has been studied primarily to determine short-term effects on respiratory and cardiovascular function. Non-painful handling associated with medical and nursing procedures have demonstrated significant physiologic destabilization. These destabilizing effects resulted in the concept of "minimal handling" which is aimed at reducing handling to the minimum necessary for the infant's survival and physical well-being. However, this concept has not been formally tested. Another important conclusion is that all types of handling, even when intended for stimulation or protection of the infant, are potentially dangerous and may unwittingly jeopardize infant health and development.

References

1. Fifer WP, Greene M, Hurtado A, Myers MM. Cardiorespiratory responses to bidirectional tilts in infants. *Early Hum Dev* 1999; 55: 265-79.

2. Mazurski JE, Birkett CL, Bedell KA, Ben-Haim SA, Segar JL. Development of baroreflex influences on heart rate variability in preterm infants. *Early Hum Dev* 1998; 53: 37-52.

3. Anthony MY, Evans DH, Levene MI. Neonatal cerebral blood flow velocity responses to changes in posture. *Arch Dis Child* 1993; 69: 304-8.

4. Schrod L, Walter J. Effect of head-up body tilt position on autonomic function and cerebral oxygenation in preterm infants. *Biol Neonate* 2002; 81: 255-9.

5. Wagaman MJ, Shutack JG, Moomjian AS, Schwartz JG, Shaffer Th, Fox WW. Improved oxygenation and lung compliance with prone positioning of neonates. *J Pediatr* 1979; 94: 787-91.

6. Martin RJ, DiFiore JM, Korenke CB, Randal H, Miller MJ, Brooks LJ. Vulnerability of respiratory control in healthy preterm infants placed supine. *Pediatrics* 1995; 127: 609-14.

7. Mizuno K, Aizawa M. Effects of body position on blood gases and lung mechanics of infants with chronic lung disease during tube feeding. *Pediatrics International* 1999; 41: 609-14.

8. Martin RJ, Herrell N, Rubin D, Fanaroff A. Effect of supine and prone positions on arterial oxygen tension in the preterm infants. *Pediatrics* 1979; 63: 528-31.

9. Baird TM, Paton JB, Fisher DE. Improved oxygenation with prone positioning in neonates: stability of increased transcutaneous pO_2. *J Perinatol* 1991; 11: 315-8.

10. McEvoy C, Mendoza ME, Bowling S, Hewlett V, Sardesai S, Durand M. Prone positioning decreases episodes of hypoxemia in extremely low birth weight infants (1000 grams or less) with chronic lung disease. *J Pediatr* 1997; 130: 305-9.

11. Heimler R, Langlois J, Hodel DJ, Nelin LD, Sasigharan P. Effect of positioning on the breathing pattern of preterm infants. *Arch Dis Child* 1992; 67: 312-4.

12. Sahni R, Schulze KF, Kashyap S, Ohira-Kist K, Fifer WP, Myers MM. Postural differences in cardiac dynamics during quiet and active sleep in low birth weight infants. *Acta Paediatr* 1999; 88: 1396-401.

13. Myers MM, Fifer WP, Schaeffer L, *et al*. Effects of sleeping position and time after feeding on the organization of sleep/wake states in prematurely born infants. *Sleep* 1998; 21: 343-9.

14. Masterson J, Zucker C, Schulze K. Prone and supine positioning effects on energy expenditure and behaviour of low birth weight neonates. *Pediatrics* 1987; 80: 689-92.

15. Goto K, Mirmiran M, Adams MM, *et al*. More awakenings and heart rate variability during supine sleep in preterm infants. *Pediatrics* 1999; 103: 603-9.

16. Kurlak LO, Ruggins NR, Stephenson TJ. Effect of nursing position on incidence, type, an duration of clinically significant apnoea in preterm infants. *Arch Dis Child* 1994; 71: F16-F19.

17. Ewer AK, James ME, Tobin JM. Prone and left lateral positioning reduce gastro-oesophageal reflux in preterm infants. *Arch Dis Child Fetal Neonatal Ed* 1999; 81: F201-F205.

18. Omar SY, Greisen G, Ibrahim MM, Youseff AM, Friis-Hansen B. Blood pressure responses to care procedures in ventilated preterm infants. *Acta Paediatr Scand* 1985; 74: 920-4.

19. Shah AR, Kurth CD, Gwiazdowski SG, Chance B, Delivoria-Papdopoulos M. Fluctuations in cerebral oxygenation and blood volume during endotracheal suctioning in premature infants. *J Pediatr* 1992; 120: 769-74.

20. Greisen G, Frederiksen PS, Hertel J, Christensen NJ. Catecholamine response to chest physiotherapy and endotracheal suctioning in preterm infants. *Acta Paediatr Scand* 1985; 74: 525-9.

21. Yeh TF, Lilien LD, Leu ST, Pildes RS. Increased oxygen consumption and energy loss in premature infants following medical care procedures. *Biol Neonate* 1984; 46: 157-62.

22. Danford DA, Miske S, Headley J, Nelson RM. Effects of routine care procedures on transcutaneous oxygen in neonates: a quantitative approach. *Arch Dis Child* 1983; 58: 20-3.

23. Mok Q, Bass CA, Ducker DA, McIntosh N. Temperature instability during nursing procedures in preterm neonates. *Arch Dis Child* 1991; 66: 783-6.

24. McCulloch KM, Ji SA, Raju TN. Skin blood flow changes during routine nursery care procedures. *Early Hum Dev* 1995; 41: 147-56.

25. Porter FL, Wolf CM, Miller P. The effect of handling and immobilization on the response to acute pain in newborn infants. *Pediatrics* 1998; 102: 1383-9.

26. Gagnon RE, Leung A, Macnab AJ. Variations in regional cerebral blood volume in neonates associated with nursery care events. *Am J Perinatol* 1999; 16: 7-11.

27. Gunnar MR, Isensee J, Fust S. Adrenocortical activity and the Brazelton Neonatal Assessment Scale: moderating effects of the newborn's biobehavioural status. *Child Dev* 1987; 58: 1448-58.

28. Porter FL, Miller PJ, Sessions Cole F, Marshall RE. A controlled clinical trial of local anesthesia for lumbar punctures in newborns. *Pediatrics* 1991; 88: 663-9.

Design and staff issues in light control

Valérie Hansen, Dominique Haumont

Neonatal care for very preterm babies has considerably improved in the last decades. The new challenge is a good quality of life for the surviving high-risk neonates. The stressful environment of the Neonatal Intensive Care Unit (NICU) itself has an impact on developmental evolution. Some long-term neurological deficits could be the consequence of inappropriate sensory stimulation for early-born neonates [1]. The visual system is the last of the sensory systems to fully develop, and is not completely mature at birth. Quite suddenly, the baby is not protected by the maternal uterus and is exposed to continuous and non-contingent bright light of the NICU. Light stimulus and overall illumination patterns in the unit might influence the way immature retina and visual function develop [2-4]. Cycled lighting regimens are more appropriate for the developmental and physiological needs of preterm neonates [5].

It is of primary importance to provide appropriate lighting conditions for fragile babies in NICUs. Individualized care also helps to accomplish this goal by systematically observing the neonate's response to interaction with the environment and adjusting the visual environment appropriately [6]. Design of future units will attend to the scientific background and current research in environmental neonatology. Lighting conditions, among other stimuli, are challenging for designers and staff working in the very particular environment of the NICU.

Design of the Neonatal Intensive Care Unit

Light and the immature visual system

The amount of light that reaches the eye depends on both physical and physiological factors [3, 4]. The basic architecture of the visual system is genetically determined. For the successful development of visual function, both endogenous stimulation, such as rapid eye movement (REM) sleep, as well as exogenous inputs are necessary. On one hand, the overall light level in the environment and the amount of light that reaches the eye is important to consider [2, 7]. On the other hand, caregiving activities, pain or other interactions with the baby alter the type and quality of REM sleep and generalized development of the neonate. All factors potentially have an impact on early visual development [8, 9].

The application of theoretical and research background to the design of a neonatal unit involves the reduction of excessive light available to the infant's eyes in the environment. Illumination levels measured in current units are often high above recommended standards [7]. NICUs are typically illuminated 24 hours a day with a mixture of daylight and artificial light. Patterns of illumination differ according to the location of the infant's bed in the nursery. Similar patterns of illumination are found at contiguous bedsides, reducing the ability to individualize lighting conditions for each baby [10]. Factors as diverse as weather conditions, location of the baby's bed, design of the unit and severity of infant's disease influence the typical amount of light at the bedside.

Guidelines for perinatal care from the American Academy of Pediatrics recommend adjustable light devices, between 10 and 600 lux (1 to 60 foot candles). Both natural and electric light sources need controls to reduce the intensity of illumination. For example, plastic filters, glass shields and dimmers may be used to control light delivered to the baby. Use of indirect lighting is recommended whenever possible [11]. Rapid darkening of the environment must also be available for transillumination and 1080 lux for procedures that necessitate direct observation and intervention. Separate lighting between adjacent beds for procedures and for support areas (medications, staff, and reception) are recommended.

Further recommendations include having one daylight source for newborn care areas, with windows glazed 2 feet (61 cm) away from baby's bed with shading devices. Patient safety has been shown not to be influenced adversely by reduced light or sound levels [12].

The level and type of light must be age appropriate. Currently, data are not conclusive regarding the effect of light on the development of retinopathy of prematurity [13]. However, regulation of infant states, REM sleep and overall growth are influenced by provision of environmental light.

A cycled-lighting regimen is more adequate (see infra) for developing infants. However, when full light is provided, lower general light levels are recommended, when compared to non-cycled regimens.

Light and circadian rhythms

Human physiology shows a circadian rhythmicity [14-18]. The endogenous circadian clock is generated from the suprachiasmatic nucleus (SCN). Input pathways relay the photic information that reaches the retina to the SCN and synchronization appears. This cycle is based on a 24-hour light-dark rhythm. Output signals are expressed by the circadian rhythms of hormones like cortisol, temperature changes, heart rate, sleep-wakefulness patterns and behaviour. In foetal life, the circadian clock is entrained by the mother's physiologic and behavioral rhythmicity. In the NICU, the early-born neonate will undergo a very different lighting environment which is typically bright and non-cycled, and which therefore does not contribute to the development of circadian rhythmicity.

Studies of Hao and Rivkees on preterm baboons showed that their biological clock was responsive to light as early as 25 weeks gestation [18]. However, Kennaway, *et al.* showed a delay in melatonin secretion in preterm compared to full term neonates [15]. Expressed circadian rhythmicity is apparently entrained by low-intensity lighting (200 lux) after birth [19]. In the absence of maternal physiologic control of circadian rhythms, it appears that the preterm infant may be readily entrained by environmental lighting. The design of the NICU must attend to those emerging physiological needs. This means a respect of the natural endogenous rhythmicity and enhancement of physiological and hormonal stability by attending to the light environment of preterm infants.

Low intensity light, especially at night, is recommended in order to have sources of daytime lighting and to adopt a cycled-light regimen in the unit. Further research is necessary to determine the ideal time of initiation of cycled lighting, and its combination with other light sources like phototherapy.

Staff issues in light control

Reduction of light levels and cycled light regimens are recommended for optimal neonatal development. Staff support is essential in the achievement of this goal. The different needs of sleeping infants and staff responsibilities must be accommodated to the best extent possible. Separate rooms with different light sources must be designed for specific tasks so that individualized lighting can be accommodated [11, 20].

Bright light is necessary for the preparation of drugs, staff rounds, and work with medical charts. Moderate levels of lighting might be more suitable for other staff responsibilities instead of a very dim light regimen. Dedicated spaces can be allocated for computer workstations within patient care areas.

Additionally, flexibility is necessary to meet the needs of their caregivers. Of course, it is essential that all individuals involved keep in mind the priorities of a good visibility, safety and accessibility to the baby. Walsh-Sukys *et al.* evaluated the impact of reducing light and sound in a level III unit [12]. Patient safety was not adversely influenced. Staff members were highly satisfied with reduction in sound levels. However, reactions to reduced light were more mixed. They led to modifications of the bedside lighting.

Substantial flexibility is required in establishing standards for lighting so that disparate needs of babies at various stages of development can be accommodated. Detailed behavioural observations that consider physiological, as well as state and motor parameters, provide a strong basis on which to assess how light and other stimuli impact the infant's stability. From these observations, an individualized developmental care program which is based on the adaptation of both the neonate's requirements and the environmental conditions can be developed. This plan of care meets the needs of babies, families and staff [9].

Relationship-based care automatically includes the neonate, parents and staff. All individuals contribute to supporting ideal neonatal development in an less than ideal environment.

Conclusion

Light stimulus for the neonate in the NICU is very different from what the foetus would have experienced in the womb. Infants in neonatal units are often exposed to a bright and continuous light environment. This exposure can be harmful for subsequent development of visual function and overall neurodevelopment. Although little is known about the impact of direct light on the retina, long term anomalies of infant visual function and infant's behaviour could be partly due to an inappropriate light environment in the NICU at the early stages of development. It is often difficult to distinguish specific effects of light among other sensory stimuli like sound, caregiving and procedures.

Light provides a great deal of information humans gain about the environment. It is based on rapid inputs to the visual system and slower inputs of information like time of day and night. The quality of light (daylight, spectrum, distribution, timing and duration) are essential tools to evaluate the impact of light in intensive care units.

There are sufficient data to recommend cycled light regimens, general reduction of light levels in the NICU to around 250 lux during the day, and reduced direct lighting. The quality of light is important as well as the opportunity to adapt the lighting intensity by special devices in case of emergency. Standards that consider the baby's and family's requirements as well as the staff's needs are necessary in attending to light recommendations.

Developmental care programs and behavioural observations offer good supports for the basic care of fragile neonates. Future research should focus on potential links between abnormal visual function and particular lighting conditions in the context of developmental caregiving. However, cycled light regimens and low levels of illumination at night are recommended from current research. The ideal age for the onset of this type of regimen is not clear at this time. From what is currently known regarding development visual function and the effects of environmental light, it is imperative that each NICU acquires acknowledge of environmental neonatology and consider its inclusion in everyday practice.

References

1. Graven SN, Bowen FW Jr, Brooten D, et al. The high-risk infant environment. The role of care giving and the social environment. *J Perinatol* 1992; 12: 267-75.

2. Lanum J. The damaging effects of light on the retina. Empirical findings, theoretical and practical implications. *Sur Ophthalmol* 1978; 22: 221-49.

3. Robinson J, Moseley MJ, Thompson JR, Fielder AR. Eyelid opening in preterm neonates. *Arch Dis Child* 1989; 64: 943-8.

4. Robinson J, Fielder AR. Light and the immature visual system. *Eye* 1992; 6: 166-72.

5. Mann NP, Haddow R, Stokes L, Goodley S, Rutter N. Effect of night and day on preterm infants in a newborn nursery. Randomised trial. *Br Med J* 1986; 293: 1265-7.

6. Als H, Lawhon G, Duffy FH, Mc Anulty GB, Gibes-Grossman R, Blickman JG. Developmental care for the very low birth weight preterm infant: Medical and neurofunctional effects. *JAMA* 1994; 272: 853-8.

7. Robinson J, Moseley MJ, Fielder AR. Illuminance of neonatal units. *Arch Dis Child* 1990; 65: 679-82.

8. Graven S. Clinical research data illuminating the relationship between the physical environment and patient medical outcomes. *J Health Des* 1997; 9: 15-9.

9. Als H, Gilkerson L. The role of relationship-based developmentally supportive newborn intensive care in strengthening outcome of preterm infants. *Semin Perinatol* 1997; 21: 178-89.

10. Fielder A, Moseley M. Environmental light and the preterm infant. *Semin Perinatol* 2000; 24: 291-8.

11. *Guidelines for Perinatal Care*, Fifth edition. Washington, DC: American Academy of Pediatrics, Elk Grove Village, Ill and American College of Obstetricians and Gynecologists, 2002.

12. Walsh-Sukys M, Reitenbach A, Hudson-Barr D, De Pompei P. Reducing light and sound in the neonatal intensive care unit: an evaluation of patient safety, staff satisfaction and costs. *J Perinatol* 2001; 21: 230-5.

13. Reynolds JD, Hardy RJ, Kennedy KA, Spencer R, van Heuven WA, Fielder AR. Lack of efficacy of light reduction in preventing retinopathy of prematurity. Light Reduction in Retinopathy of Prematurity (LIGHT-ROP) Cooperative Group. *N Engl J Med* 1998; 338: 1572-6.

14. Mirmiran M, Ariagno R. Influence of light in the NICU and development of circadian rhythms in preterm infants. *Semin Perinatol* 2000; 24: 247-57.

15. Kennaway D, Stamp G, Goble F. Development of melatonin production in infants and the impact of prematurity. *J Clin Endocrinol Metab* 1992; 75: 367-9.

16. Miller CL, White R, Whitman TL, O'Callaghan MF, Maxwell S. The effect of cycled versus non-cycled lighting on the growth and development of preterm infants. *Infant Behav Dev* 1995; 18: 95-102.

17. Rivkees S. Developing circadian rhythmicity. Basic and clinical aspects. *Pediatr Clin North Am* 1997; 44: 467-87.

18. Hao H, Rivkees SA. The biological clock of very premature primates infants is responsive to light. *Proc Natl Acad Sci USA* 1999; 96: 2426-9.

19. McGraw K, Hoffmann R, Harker C, Herman JH. The development of circadian rhythms in a human infant. *Sleep* 1999; 22: 303-10.

20. Shepley MM. Pre-design and postoccupancy analysis of staff behaviour in a neonatal intensive care unit. *Child Health Care* 2002; 31: 237-53.

Developmental care:
A breast-feeding perspective

Kerstin Hedberg Nyqvist

Human beings are mammals

Numerous factors are important for approaching "normalcy" in the infant's daily life in spite of an initial need of neonatal care. Breast-feeding should be regarded as a core aspect of this "normalcy" a practice related to the provision of medical and nursing care, and a part of the infant's social and physical environment. In consideration of breast-feeding being an aspect of "normalcy", it is important to bear in mind that human beings are mammals. Mammals are characterized as a species by secreting a fluid that serves as sole nutrition for their young. Among mammals, there is a correlation between length of gestation, age at onset of puberty, length of life, and duration of breast-feeding of several years. – With small marsupials at one end of the continuum, and primates at the other extreme of the continuum [1, 2]. Breast-feeding patterns are also found in primates. The young chimpanzee suckles several times per hour. The chimpanzee mother sleeps with and nurses its young at night.

Some of the mammalian human descendants of primates still live in hunting-gathering and agricultural societies. Breast-feeding by these human descendants occurs frequently (an average of four feeds per hour) with feeds equally distributed over a 24-hour period, and characteristically continues for 2 to 6 years. In humans, length of gestation, age at onset of puberty, and length of life is longer than in the other primates. In nonindustrialized societies, the predominant feeding pattern is demand breast-feeding, and the infants have constant access to the mother's breast, even at night. Children are weaned at 2-3 years of age or later. In industrialized countries this pattern was "rediscovered" when researchers found that increased nursing frequency resulted in increased milk production [3].

In spite of the human history as mammals where mother-infant early contact was essential to survival, mother-infant separation after birth was institutionalized in industrialized countries, resulting in lower breast-feeding rates. For full term healthy infants, the Baby Friendly Hospitals Initiative has reversed this trend. For preterm and sick infants, however, the situation is very different from the normal uninterrupted mother-infant contact after birth.

The current goal for breast-feeding, as defined by the World Health Assembly, is exclusive breast-feeding for 6 months and continuation of breast-feeding after introduction of other foods during the infant's first two years of life and beyond [4]. In European countries, there is a wide variation in breast-feeding initiation and duration rates [5]. Breast-feeding data for preterm infants are scarce and predominantly consist of reports of small samples. A Swedish study found no significant difference in breast-feeding initiation rate between low birth weight (LBW) infants and full term infants, but noted shorter breast-feeding duration among the LBW infants [6].

Benefits of breast-milk and breast-feeding

In addition to being the ideal nutrition for preterm infants, breast-milk has been described as the proximal mechanism for behavioral change in newborn mammals [7]. Breast-feeding activates the endogenous opiod system that plays an important role in reorganizing activity, altering sensory responsiveness and supporting associative learning. It may be hypothesized that similar mechanisms are present in human infants.

The first period of a human infant's life can be regarded as an external continuation of the pregnancy, as the infant depends on contact with the mother for a harmonious adaptation to extrauterine life. Therefore, ingestion of nourishment is definitely not the sole purpose of mother-infant interaction when the infant is positioned at the mother's breast. Breast-feeding supports an infant's developmental tasks in exploring himself and the world. It helps the infant to discriminate signals from the social and physical environment and to respond appropriately while maintaining physiologic and behavioral stability. Breast-feeding provides the infant with multimodal stimulation: tactile, auditory, visual, thermal, gustatory, olfactory, vestibular, and proprioceptive, additionally supporting the development of a normal diurnal rhythm. The infant's early touch of the mother's nipple seems to have positive influence on the mother-infant relationship as well [8]. The amount of dyadic experience after birth affects the quality of interaction between mothers and their preterm infants [9]. Mothers' breast-feeding experiences are related to specific emotional advantages. It has been suggested that lack of affectionate body-to-body contact in preterm infants may lead to symptoms of "reactive attachment disorder" [10].

A meta-analysis of cognitive function in breast- and formula fed children showed significant differences, with sustained effects through 15 years of age, even after adjustment for socioeconomic variables and maternal education [11]. In LBW infants, these differences were even greater. Lucas [12] showed a dose-response relationship between the proportion of breast milk in the diet and subsequent intelligence quotients (IQ) in infants who were born preterm. Components of breast milk that are of particular importance are the long-chain fatty acids docosahexanoic acid (DHA) and arachidonic acid (AA). These elements are found in the brain, retina, and red cell membranes, and contribute to neurological development and visual acuity. Breast milk is a carrier of other multiple biochemical and immunological messages (hormones, growth factors, cytokines, secretory IgA, lactoferrin, lysozyme, oligosaccharides) that influence gastrointestinal development and host defense mechanisms. Enhanced protection against infections have been documented several years after the termination of breast-feeding [13, 14]. One mechanism for host defenses is the enteromammary system, activated by mother-infant physical contact in the neonatal unit and mediated by immunoglobulins on the mother's milk.

Hospital practices

As a result of the WHO/UNICEF Baby Friendly Hospitals Initiative (BFHI), newborn healthy infants normally enjoy uninterrupted contact with their mothers, and breast-feeding commences immediately after birth. However, as pointed out by Levin in his program for "humane neonatal care" [15], the BFHI program does not address neonatal intensive care units. Preterm and sick newborn infants are commonly deprived of the normal psychosocial environment – their mother's body. Instead, they are exposed to a disturbing physical environment and to procedures that cause considerable discomfort and pain. In spite of the benefits of breast milk, restrictive guidelines are still common regarding introduction of breast-feeding and advancement of oral feeding in preterm infants. In industrialized countries, a postmenstrual age of around 34 weeks has been commonly established for the commencement of breast-feeding. Conflicting practices and advice regarding breast-feeding are common causes of complaint by mothers.

An intervention that is based on mother-infant skin-to-skin contact and breast-feeding is the Kangaroo Mother Care (KMC) method, which was first established in Colombia in order to reduce infant mortality and morbidity [16]. Since then, the method has been implemented in all types of settings with numerous studies of its effects having been conducted. KMC is defined as "early, prolonged and continuous (as allowed by circumstances) skin-to-skin contact between the mother and her newborn low birth weight infant, ideally with exclusive breast-feeding. It is recommended both in the hospital and after adequately supported early (depending on local circumstances) discharge and follow-up, until at least the 40th week of postnatal gestational age" [17]. Effects of KMC include lower rates of severe illness, improved prevalence and duration of breast-feeding, improved thermal control, physiologic stability, enhanced sleep organization, and shorter hospital stays. Mothers have described feelings of healing from the crisis of premature birth as an effect of skin-to-skin contact with their infants [18]. Changes in mothers' perception of their infants and increased confidence in the maternal role have also been noted [19]. In order to facilitate safe implementation of the KMC method, the WHO published a practical guide for the method in 2003 [20].

Sucking capacity in preterm infants

Conflicting policies for breast-feeding in KMC programs in low-income countries and restrictive guidelines in industrialized countries became the impetus for a study of KMC in Uppsala, Sweden. The only criteria for commencing breast-feeding in the study was that the infant had been weaned off ventilator and Continuous Positive Airway Pressure (CPAP), and did not show signs of fragility such as severe apnoea, bradycardia or oxygen desaturations in connection with handling. Breast-feeding was introduced from 27 weeks postmenstrual age (PMA) with 71 infants born at 26-35 weeks of gestation [21, 22]. Mothers received weekly guidance about interaction with their infant in connection with breast-feeding according to the Newborn Individualized Developmental Care and Assessment Program (NIDCAP) model [23]. The infant's breast-feeding behavior was recorded throughout the infant's hospital stay according to the Preterm Infant Breastfeeding Behavior Scale (PIBBS) [24]. The PIBBS is a method for direct observation by mothers and professionals of infant competence in rooting, areolar grasp, duration of staying fixed at the breast, sucking behavior, and swallowing. On the first day with breast-feeding, all infants with data showed rooting behavior, latched on to the breast and sucked, irrespective of the infant's current post menstrual age (PMA). Nutritive sucking (defined as intake of > 5 ml verified by test weighing) was noted from 30 weeks PMA. Sixty-seven infants (94%) were breastfed at discharge, 57 (80%) of them were fully breastfed. Full breast-feeding was attained at a mean of 36.0 (33.4-40.0) weeks. Earlier birth and thus short gestation was associated with earlier development of oral motor competence [25]. Infants with a longer period of ventilator support and additional oxygen attained full breast-feeding at a later maturational level. This early ability may be interpreted to be a result of learning experience, elicited and enhanced by contingent stimuli in a developmentally supportive environment.

Developmentally supportive breast-feeding interventions

The following interventions are recommended for inclusion in policies and programs for breast-feeding support in neonatal care:

1. Early introduction and advancement of enteral feeds (preferably with the mother's expressed milk and/or donor breast milk).

2. Early initiation of regular breast milk expression day and night.

3. A strategy for decreasing mother-infant separation: providing rooms for mothers in the neonatal unit for living-in and rooming-in, merging maternity units and neonatal units, and offering neonatal care in the home.

4. Skin-to-skin contact between mothers (and fathers) and their infants while receiving ventilator treatment as soon as tolerated.

5. Application of the KMC method according to the WHO guidelines, as allowed by the infant's medical condition and the circumstances.

6. Encouragement of initiation of breast-feeding with the infants' medical stability as the only criterion, irrespective of gestational age at birth, current postmenstrual or postnatal age, or weight, or any other criterion.

7. Application of the NIDCAP model for guidance to mothers regarding interaction with their infants during breast-feeding. A case report of an infant girl at a PMA of 29 weeks using NIDCAP observations during breast-feeding documented several differences in both maternal behavior as well as the infant's physiologic stability, motor behavior, level of alertness, and sucking behavior. These differences were noted before and after guidance to the mother about interaction based on the infant's behavioral cues [23]. The recommendations offered to this mother after an initial

NIDCAP observation included holding the infant in a flexor position with still hands, shielding the infant's face from direct light, and reducing multi-modal stimulation such as simultaneous talking and rocking. During the second observation, after the mother modified her behavior, the infant showed repeated active sucking during 15 minutes of breast-feeding, frequent smiling, and she ingested 11 millilitres of milk.

8. Provide guidance to mothers in how to observe their infant at the breast according to the PIBBS. This method facilitate assessment of the mother's and infant's need for improved positioning and interventions for encouraging rooting, latching-on to the breast, staying fixed at the breast, and more active sucking. Examples of maternal interactive behavior are shown in *table I*.

Table I. Maternal behavior during breast-feeding.

Functioning interaction	Problematic interaction
Positions the infant at the breast at signs of higher behavioral state (waking up, awake), at discrete interest in signs of sucking.	Positions the infant at the breast when he is asleep and continues to try to wake up the infant in spite of lack of signs of interest in sucking.
Selects a quiet place where the infant is shielded from bright light, noise, activity and visual input.	Selects a place with bright light, noise, activity and visual input.
Sits in an upright position.	Sits in a reclining position.
Places the infant on a pillow, etc. Gives support to a straight infant trunk position. Supports infant's head in a position directed forwards; the mouth is in front of the nipple.	Holds the infant with inadequate support, the infant's trunk is not straight, the head is not directed forwards, and the mouth is not in front of the nipple.
Places the infant with arms and legs flexed, using her clothes for support and protection from cold stress.	Holds the infant with extended arms and legs, does not cover the infant.
Gives consistent support for a correct position with still hands.	Moves her hands, changes the infant's position often, inadequate support.
Offers the infant the breast by gently touching the infant's lips with the nipple to elicit rooting.	Opens the infant's mouth, inserts the nipple into the infant's mouth.
When the infant does not respond: lets him rest, waits for signs of interest in sucking/alertness.	Continues her efforts to make the infant latch on in spite of no response.
At signs if rooting, pulls the infant closer to her body, with the nose touching the breast and the chin "pressed into" the breast.	Holds the infant loosely, at some distance from her body, nose and chin do not touch the breast.
Focuses her attention mainly at the infant. Does not seem to pay much interest in the environment.	Focuses her attention at the environment, looks occasionally at the infant.
Has a relaxed face.	Seems worried, uncomfortable, bored.
Is attentive to the infant's position at the breast and makes appropriate adjustments when needed.	Does not notice incorrect position, makes no adjustments.
When the infant makes long pauses during sucking: encourages sucking by talking or gently depressing breast tissue in front of the infant's nose to achieve stimulation of the sucking reflex by touching the hard palate – in case of no response: gives time-out.	Does not stimulate sucking, or stimulates the infant repeatedly by tickling face and body, rocking, talking, moving the breast, or repositioning. Does not notice lack of response.
Is mainly quiet, may talk sometimes in a soft voice with infant's father, staff, other parents.	Talks in a loud voice with staff, infant's father, staff other parents.
Lets the infant suck until he stops sucking or or lets go of the breast.	Interrupts or terminates breast-feeding while the infant is sucking.

9. The use of cups instead of bottles as an alternative oral feeding method during the transition from tube feeding to breast-feeding. Introduction of cup feeding has resulted in increased breast-feeding rates [26] and is feasible from a postmenstrual age of 30 weeks [27]. Another model associated with higher likelihood of breast-feeding, is transitioning from tube to breast feeding with nasogastric supplementation instead of bottle feeding [28].

10. A modified demand feeding schedule with a minimum number of feeds per 24 hours. The mother places the infant to the breast at the slightest sign of alertness, and – when required – places the infant at the breast also when he is asleep in order to offer opportunities for waking up and sucking and thereby reach an appropriate number of suckling episodes.

11. Education of professionals in NIDCAP and in research-based practices for support of lactation and breast-feeding in neonatal care.

References

1. Kennel JH. Keynote address: The human and health significance of parent-infant contact. *J Am Osteopath Assoc* 1987; 87: 638-45.

2. Nelson AES. Child care practices in nonindustrialized societies. *Pediatrics* 2000; 105: e75.

3. De Carvalho M. Robertson S, Friedman A, Klaus M. Effect of frequent breast-feeding on early milk production and infant weight gain. *Pediatrics* 1982; 72: 307-11.

4. WHO, UNICEF. *Global strategy on Infant and young child feeding.* Geneva: WHO, 2003. ISBN 92 4 156221 8.

5. Yngve A, Sjostrom M. Breastfeeding in countries of the European Union and EFTA: Current and proposed recommendations, rationale, prevalence, duration and trends. *Public Health Nutr* 2001; 4: 631-45.

6. Flacking R, Nyqvist KH, Ewald U, Wallin L. Long-term duration of breast-feeding in Swedish low birth weight infants. *J Hum Lact* 2003; 19: 157-65.

7. Smotherman WP, Robinson SR. Milk as the proximal mechanism for behavioral change in the newborn. *Acta Paediatr Supplement* 1994; 397: 64-70.

8. Widstrom AM, Wahlberg V, Matthiesen AS, *et al.* Short-term effects of early suckling and touch of the nipple on maternal behavior. *Early Hum Dev* 1990; 21: 153-63.

9. Eizirik LS, Bohlin G, Hagekull B. Interaction between mother and preterm infant at 34 weeks post-conceptional age. *Early Development and Parenting* 1994; 3: 171-80.

10. Goodfriend MS. Treatment of attachment disorder of infancy in a neonatal intensive care unit. *Pediatrics* 1993; 91: 139-42.

11. Anderson JW, Johnstone BM, Remley DT. Breast-feeding and cognitive development: A meta-analysis. *Am J Clin Nutr* 1999; 70: 525-35.

12. Lucas A. Morley R, Cole TJ. Randomized trial of early diet in preterm babies and later intelligence quotient. *BMJ* 1998; 317: 1481-7.

13. Hanson LA. The mother-offspring dyad and the immune system. *Acta Paediatr* 2000; 89: 252-8.

14. Schanler RJ, Hurst NM, Lau V. The use of human milk and breast-feeding in premature Infants. *Clin Perinatol* 1999; 26: 379-98.

15. Levin A. Humane neonatal care initiative. *Acta Paediatr* 1999; 88: 353-5.

16. Gomez HM, Sanabria ER, Marquette CM. The mother kangaroo programme. *Int Child Health* 1992; 3: 55-67.

17. Cattaneo A, Davanzo R, Uxa F, Tamburlini G for the International Network on Kangaroo Mother Care. Recommendations for the implementation of Kangaroo Mother Care for low birthweight infants. *Acta Paediatr* 1998; 87: 440-5.

18. Affonso D, Bosque E, Wahlberg V, Brady JP. Reconciliation and healing for mothers through skin-to-skin contact provided in an American tertiary level intensive care nursery. *Neonatal Netw* 1993; 12: 25-32.

19. Tessier R, Christo M, Velez S, *et al.* Kangaroo mother care and the bonding hypothesis. *Pediatrics* 1998; 102 (2): e17.

20. WHO. *Kangaroo mother care. A practical guide. Department of Reproductive Health and Research.* Geneva: WHO, 2003. ISBN 92 4 159035 1.

21. Nyqvist KH, Ewald U, Sjödén P-O. Development of preterm infants' breast-feeding behavior. *Early Hum Dev* 1999; 55: 247-64.

22. Nyqvist KH. The development of preterm infants' milk intake during breast feeding. *Journal of Neonatal Nursing* 2001; 7: 48-52.

23. Nyqvist KH, Ewald U, Sjödén P-O. Supporting a preterm infant's behavior during breast-feeding: A case report. *J Hum Lact* 1996; 12: 221-8.

24. Nyqvist KH, Rubertsson C, Ewald U, Sjödén P-O. Development of the preterm infant breast-feeding behavior scale (PIBBS), a study of nurse-mother agreement. *J Hum Lact* 1996; 12: 207-19.

25. Nyqvist KH, Ewald U. Infant and maternal factors in the development of breast-feeding behavior and breast-feeding outcome in preterm infants. *Acta Paediatr* 1999; 88: 1194-203.

26. Jones E. Breastfeeding in preterm infants. *Mod Midwife* 1994; 22-6.

27. Malhotra N, Vishwambaran L, Sundaram KR, Narayanan I. A controlled trial of alternative methods of oral feeding in neonates. *Early Hum Dev* 1999: 54: 29-38.

28. Klithermes PA, Cross ML, Lanese MG, Johnson KM, Simon SD. Transitioning preterm infants with nasogastric tube supplementation: Increased likelihood of breast-feeding. *JOGNN* 1999; 28: 264-73.

Now more immature preterm infants have been included in studies of skin-to-skin care. For the majority of preterm infants who weigh less than 1500 grams, skin-to-skin holding does not result in hypothermia or an increase in oxygen consumption [27, 28]. Only preterm infants with a gestational age below 27 weeks had unstable body temperature when skin-to-skin holding was done within the first week of life [29]. Skin-to-skin holding of ventilated preterm infants has been reported [30], but the transfer of the ventilated infant from the incubator to the mother resulted in physiologic instability. Therefore, this practice cannot be recommended until information about the benefit-risk ratio of this intervention for this very unstable group of patients is available.

Reported benefits of skin-to-skin holding are improved breast-feeding [24, 31] and improved weight gain [25]. Skin-to-skin holding is associated with a high degree of mother satisfaction and improves mothers' emotional adjustment after preterm delivery [32]. Even mothers of extremely immature, but spontaneously breathing preterm infants (gestational age 27-30 weeks) perceive skin-to-skin contact with their infants as a positive and helpful intervention when they participate in skin-to-skin contact regularly and for increasing duration within the first two postnatal weeks [33]. During skin-to-skin holding of ventilated preterm infants, however, parental apprehensions are a relevant problem [34].

Skin-to-skin care has several aspects that support the infant's neurobehavioural development. It promotes stability of heart and respiratory function, it is a time when the infant is protected from painful interventions, it offers opportunity for maternal proximity and interaction, and provides stimulation by skin-to-skin contact, stroking, and by the sound of the mother's body and voice. Reported short-term benefits are an increase in sleep time [29, 35, 36]. Yet there are few studies of medium-term or long-term effects of skin-to-skin holding on neurodevelopment [37].

Conclusions and directions for future research

Positioning and handling are of particular interest with the implementation of developmental care and skin-to-skin holding in the neonatal intensive care units. Positioning and handling procedures are regarded not only as means to protect fragile infants from excessive sensory input but also an opportunity to support infants' neurodevelopment. Positional support is used to prevent postural deformities and to facilitate state regulation. Non-painful handling necessary for the care and physical well-being of preterm infants, is modified to include periods of rest, to include consolation after stressful experiences and synchronized with the infant's sleep-wake cycle. Skin-to-skin holding has the additional advantage of supporting intensive involvement of parents in the care of their preterm infant. It is a period of rest, protection and close interaction between infants and their parents.

This review indicates that the techniques of positioning and handling can be of benefit for preterm infants. However, the results reported are based on studies with methodological difficulties: (1) Techniques of positioning and handling are studied within the framework of protocols including multiple interventions. Therefore it is difficult to evaluate the benefit of the individual procedure. (2) Long-term data confirming the persistence of reported short-term benefits on neurodevelopment are not yet available. (3) Studies usually are small and use a broad variety of measures making clinical significance difficult to interpret.

Therefore, future studies could address the effect of clearly specified single interventions on major clinical and long-term developmental outcomes. Additionally, they should define the populations of preterm infants who might benefit most from positioning and handling interventions.

References

1. Task Force on infant sleep position and sudden infant death syndrome. Changing concepts of sudden infant death syndrome: implications for infant sleeping environment and sleep position. *Pediatrics* 2000; 105: 650-6.

2. Oyen N, Markestad T, Skjaerven R, *et al*. Combined effects of sleeping position and prenatal risk factors in sudden infant death syndrome: The Nordic Epidemiology SIDS Study. *Pediatrics* 1997; 100: 613-21.

3. Adams MM, Kugener B, Mirmiran M, Ariagno RL. Survey of sleeping position after hospital discharge in healthy preterm infants. *J Perinatol* 1998; 18: 168-72.

4. Martin RJ, DiFiore JM, Korenke CB, Randal H, Miller MJ, Brooks LJ. Vulnerability of respiratory control in healthy preterm infants placed supine. *Pediatrics* 1995; 127: 609-14.

5. Constantin E, Waters KA, Morielli A, Brouillette RT. Head turning and face-down positioning in prone-sleeping premature infants. *J Pediatr* 1999; 134: 558-62.

6. Bhat RY, Leipälä JA, Rafferty GF, Hannam S, Greenough A. Survey of sleeping position recommendations for prematurely born infants on neonatal intensive care unit discharge. *Eur J Pediatr* 2003; 162: 426-7.

7. Davis BE, Moon RY, Sachs HC, Ottolini MC. Effects of sleep position on infant motor development. *Pediatrics* 1998; 102: 1135-40.

8. Konishi Y, Kuriyama M, Mikawa H, Suzuki J. Effect of body position on later postural and functional lateralities of preterm infants. *Dev Med Child Neurol* 1987; 29: 751-7.

9. Jenni OG, vonSiebenthal K, Wolf M, Keel M, Duc G, Bucher HU. Effect of nursing in the head elevated tilt position (15°) on the incidence of bradycardic and hypoxemic episodes in preterm infants. *Pediatrics* 1997; 100: 622-5.

10. Fearon I, Kisilevski BS, Hains SM, Muir DW, Tranmer J. Swaddling after heel lance: age-specific effects on behavioural recovery in preterm infants. *J Dev Behav Pediatr* 1997; 18: 222-32.

11. Neu M, Browne JV. Infant physiologic and behavioural organization during swaddled versus unswaddled weighing. *J Perinatol* 1997; 17: 193-8.

12. Short MA, Brooks-Brunn JA, Reeves DS, Yeager J, Thorpe JA. The effects of swaddling versus standard positioning on neuromuscular development in very low birth weight infants. *Neonatal Network* 1996; 15: 2-31.

13. Beckman CA. Use of neonatal boundaries to improve outcomes. *J Holist Nurs* 1997; 15: 54-67.

14. Davies PM, Robinson R, Harris L, Cartlidge PH. Persistent mild hip deformation in preterm infants. *Arch Dis Child* 1993; 69: 597-8.

15. Downs JA, Edwards AD, McCormick DC, Roth SC, Stewart AL. Effect of intervention on development of hip posture in very preterm babies. *Arch Dis Child* 1991; 66: 797-801.

16. Monterosso L, Kristjanson LJ, Cole J, Evans SF. Effect of postural supports on neuromotor function in very preterm infants to term equivalent age. *J Paediatr Child Health* 2003; 39: 197-205.

17. Stening W, Nitsch P, Wassmer G, Roth B. Cardiorespiratory stability of premature and term infants carried in infant slings. *Pediatrics* 2002; 110: 879-83.

18. Speidel BD. Adverse effects of routine procedures on preterm infants. *The Lancet* 1978; 2: 864-6.

19. Langer VS. Minimal handling protocol for the intensive care nursery. *Neonatal Network* 1990; 9: 23-7.

20. Als H, Lawhon G, Brown E, et al. Individualized behavioural and environmental care for the very low-birth-weight preterm infant at high risk for bronchopulmonary dysplasia: neonatal intensive care unit and developmental outcome. *Pediatrics* 1986; 78: 1123-32.

21. Als H, Lawhon G, Duffy FH, McAnulty GB, Gibes-Grossman R, Blickman JG. Individualized developmental care for the very low-birth-weight preterm infant. *JAMA* 1994; 272: 853-8.

22. Cole J, Begish-Duddy A, Judas ML, Jorgensen KM. Changing the NICU environment: the Boston City Hospital model. *Neonatal Network* 1990; 9: 15-23.

23. Charpak N, Ruiz-Pelaez JG, Charpak Y. Rey-Martinez Kangaroo mother program: an alternative way of caring of low birth weight infants? One year mortality in a two cohort study. *Pediatrics* 1994; 94: 804-10.

24. Whitelaw A, Heisterkamp G, Sleath K, Acolet D, Richards M. Skin to skin contact for very low birth weight infants and their mothers. *Arch Dis Child* 1988; 63: 1377-81.

25. Wahlberg V, Affonso DD, Pearson B. A retrospective, comparative study using the kangaroo method as a complement to the standard incubator care. *Eur J Public Health* 1992; 2: 34-7.

26. Ludington-Hoe SM, Thompson C, Swinth J, Hadeed AJ, Anderson GC. Kangaroo Care: research results, and practice implications and guidelines. *Neonatal Network* 1994; 13: 19-27.

27. Bauer J, Sontheimer D, Fischer C, Linderkamp O. Metabolic rate and energy balance in very low birth weight infants during kangaroo holding by their mothers and fathers. *J Pediatr* 1996; 129: 608-11.

28. Bauer K, Uhrig C, Sperling P, Pasel K, Wieland C, Versmold HT. Body temperatures and oxygen consumption during skin-to-skin (kangaroo) care in stable preterm infants weighing less than 1500 g. *J Pediatr* 1997; 130: 240-4.

29. Bauer K, Pyper A, Sperling P, Uhrig C, Versmold H. Effects of gestational and postnatal age on body temperature, oxygen consumption, and activity during early skin-to-skin contact between preterm infants of 25-30-week gestation and their mothers. *Pediatr Res* 1998; 44: 247-51.

30. Ludington-Hoe SM, Ferreira CN, Goldstein MR. Kangaroo care with a ventilated preterm infant. *Acta Paediatr* 1998; 87: 711-6.

31. Blaymore Bier JA, Ferguson AE, Morales Y, et al. Comparison of skin-to-skin contact with standard contact in low-birth-weight infants who are breast-fed. *Arch Pediatr Adolesc Med* 1996; 150: 1265-9.

32. Affonso DD, Wahlberg V, Persson B. Exploration of mother's reactions to the kangaroo method of prematurity care. *Neonatal Network* 1989; 7: 43-51.

33. Bauer K, Uhrig C, Versmold H. Maternal perception of early skin-to-skin contact with their very immature preterm infants of 27-30 weeks gestation. *Z Geburtsh Neonatol* 1999; 203: 250-4.

34. Neu M. Parents' perception of skin-to-skin care with their preterm infants requiring assisted ventilation. *J Obstet Gynecol Neonatal Nurs* 1999; 28: 157-64.

35. Messmer PR, Rodriguez S, Adams J, et al. Effect of kangaroo care on sleep time for neonates. *Pediatr Nurs* 1997; 23: 408-14.

36. Feldman R, Eidelman AI. Skin-to-skin contact (Kangoroo Care) accelerates automonic and neurobehavioural maturation in preterm infants. *Dev Med Child Neurol* 2003; 45: 274-81.

37. Feldman R, Eidelman AI, Sirota L, Weller A. Comparison of skin-to-skin (kangaroo) and traditional care: parenting outcomes and preterm infant development. *Pediatrics* 2002; 110: 16-26.

Non-pharmacological pain control in neonates

Véronique Pierrat, Nathalie Goubet, Cécile Rattaz, Thierry Debillon

In the past 15 years, neonates' ability to perceive and react to pain has been acknowledged [1, 2]. There has been increasing focus among neonatal researchers on the study of expression of pain in preterm and full-term neonates, on analysis of its developmental impact, and on the investigation of alleviation of pain. These perspectives and studies have provided a wealth of data. It is now widely accepted that neonates receiving intensive care, should receive central analgesics, administered intravenously to relieve pain.

Routine, invasive procedures are frequent in the most immature infants [3]. However, because there is concern about the adverse effects of pharmacological interventions, application in daily routine medical care of newborns has been limited. Although knowledge on non-pharmacological pain alleviation has improved considerably, routine care is still being done without significant behavioral pain management. Consequently the challenge of providing simple, safe, and effective pain-relieving interventions for neonates is still an ongoing dilemma in most neonatal units.

In this paper, we will review the non-pharmacological methods to alleviate pain. Recent research suggests that a multivariate approach including physiological, behavioural and contextual indices could be the most valid measure of pain [5], although physiological and behavioral can be highly correlated and as a result may be redundant [6]. We will not deal with the specific issue of measuring pain in neonates, although it is a related and important topic [4]. Our review of the literature will also not distinguish between multivariate and univariate approaches to non-pharmacologic pain management.

Environmental and behavioral strategies

Thanks to the early work of Als and colleagues [7], it has been recognized that infants in the NICU are exposed to a multitude of extremely noxious stimuli [8-10]. These include bright lights, loud sounds, frequent handling, and repeated painful procedures. Such a noxious environment results in physiologic and behavioral disorganization, which in turns alters responses to pain.

Recent studies [11, 12] have shown that neonates' pain responses are influenced by the number of painful procedures previously experienced by the infant, and the length of time since the last procedure. The most complex and exhaustive program designed to modify the preterm newborn's physical and human environment is the Newborn Individualized Developmental Care and Assessment Program (NIDCAP) described by Als [13]. Most of the procedures used in this program as strategies for preventing neonatal pain have been reviewed by Franck and Lawhon [14]. The NIDCAP method provides a preventive and integrative approach for minimizing neonatal discomfort by promoting the infant's own regulatory capacities to cope with stress. However, not all of its aspects have been validated.

Reducing noxious stimuli in the environment

The most obvious strategy to decrease pain is to limit invasive testing and invasive care. This does not deserve validation and appears to be one of the first steps to take. Furthermore, reducing noxious stimuli promotes infants' physiological and behavioral stability [5, 15] and may reduce pain. In addition, improved coordination of care can help to minimize pain during invasive procedures. Porter [6] has shown that newborns who received a heel stick shortly after having undergone handling displayed increased pain reactions compared to newborns who were left undisturbed before the heel stick.

Containing and positioning

Swaddling the infant in a blanket, combined with vestibular interventions like rocking has been effective in promoting stability in physiological indicators and behavioral states in the newborn [16]. Several other studies have shown the efficacy of swaddling [17] or rocking [18] to minimize crying and physiological changes after a heel stick. In a recent study, Gray and colleagues [19] showed that skin-to-skin contact was a remarkably potent intervention against pain experienced during heel stick in a group of 30 healthy full-term newborns. This single procedure reduced crying by 82% and grimacing by 65% compared to a control group.

Choice of the blood sampling method

Heel sticks are the conventional method of blood sampling in neonates. It is easy to perform and done by the nursing staff in most countries. By contrast, venipuncture can be performed either by nurses or by the medical staff. The choice of the method is important with regards to pain. The pain response and acceptability by parents was found to be better with venipuncture than with heel stick [20, 21]. The distress associated with heel pricks can be lowered by the use of spring loading lance [22, 23]. Recently, Eriksson [24] found that if oral glucose is given prior to skin puncture (either heel stick or venipuncture), the choice of blood sampling method has no impact on pain symptoms in full term babies.

Non-nutritive sucking

Non-nutritive sucking during heel lance substantially reduces crying and grimacing [25] and blunts heart rate increases [26] in preterm and term newborns. When compared to swaddling [27], rocking [18] or even sweet solutions [28], pacifiers soothed infants more rapidly. Franck [29] reported that neonatal nurses ranked a pacifier as their first choice to manage pain. It is a simple, cost-effective way of calming infants, although there is a debate among those who promote breast feeding in the light of some studies suggesting that pacifiers are contra-indicated for breast feeding term babies [30].

Sucrose

The analgesic effect of sucrose has been the most frequently studied non-pharmacologic intervention for relief of procedural pain in neonates [31-37]. A study performed by Carbajal [38] compared the analgesic effects of sucrose, glucose and pacifiers in term neonates. Pacifiers alone were more effective than sweet solutions to decrease the behavioral responses associated with pain, and the effects of 30% sucrose and 30% glucose were equivalent. Furthermore, the association of sucrose with a pacifier showed a trend towards lower pain scores compared with pacifiers alone.

Recently, the efficacy of sucrose has been systematically reviewed in two meta-analyses [39, 40]. The results indicate that sucrose does reduce procedural pain in neonates. The optimal dose could not be identified, but very small doses of 24% sucrose (0.01-0.02 g) have been reported to reduce pain in very low birth weight infants. In term infants, larger doses (0.24 to 0.50 g) given by syringe or pacifier approximately 2 min prior to a painful stimulus were the most effective in diminishing proportion of cry. However, data about efficacy and side-effects are lacking. Recently Johnston [41] suggested that repeated use of sucrose analgesia in infants < 31 weeks' PCA may put infants at risk for poorer neurobehavioral development and physiologic outcomes. The association of sucrose with rocking was tested in two studies [42, 43]. In a population of preterm infants born between 25 and 34 weeks post-conceptual age, Johnston [42] was unable to show a positive effect of simulated rocking alone on facial expressions and heart rate after a heel prick. Sucrose combined with simulated rocking tended to be more effective than sucrose alone [42, 43].

Other sweet solutions

As sucrose is not widely used in neonatal units, others sweet solutions like glucose or breast milk have been tested [38, 44-46]. In these studies, glucose [38, 46] or solutions containing glucose [44] with a concentration of at least 30% seem to be as effective as sucrose to alleviate pain. Glucose (30%) has been shown to be more effective in reducing symptoms associated with pain for venipuncture than local anesthetic cream EMLA® [47]. In very preterm neonates, a small dose of 0.3 ml of 30% glucose has an analgesic effect during subcutaneous injections [37]. However the synergistic analgesic effect of glucose plus a pacifier was less obvious in this population as opposed to what other studies have shown in full-term neonates. Breast feeding can also effectively reduce response to pain during minor invasive procedure in term neonates [48, 49]. It is at least as effective as that observed with 30% glucose plus sucking a pacifier [49].

Familiar odor

Olfaction is thought to be an important aspect of the human experience for its role in emotional, cognitive and social development. Recently, the calming effect of a familiar odor following a painful procedure was demonstrated by Rattaz et al. [50]. In a group of 44 full-term infants, they showed that a familiar odor (mother's milk odor or familiar vanilla) presented during and after a heel stick led to quicker recovery after the invasive procedure was over. Moreover, infants exposed to their mother's milk odor during the heel sticks displayed less agitation. The familiar odor did not alleviate pain during the procedure itself, but allowed the baby to self-regulate and calm down after the procedure. This effect is different from sucrose, pacifiers and skin-to-skin contact in that the familiar odor does not provide analgesia, but it provides comfort after the invasive procedure is over, as swaddling does. In a related study with preterm infants, Goubet and colleagues [51] showed that smelling a familiar odor during a venipuncture prevented premature newborns from mounting a full blown pain response. By contrast, smelling a familiar odor during a heel stick, a more painful procedure, led to a decrease in pain reactions after the heel stick was over but not during the procedure. The effect of the familiar odor seems to have been mediated by the baby's previous experience with the odor because an unfamiliar odor was not soothing. The soothing effect cannot be explained as a mobilization of infants' attentional resources but its familiarity seems to be the key factor.

It is of interest to note that we now have evidence that all three components of the nursing-suckling behavior – contact, suckling, and taste/flavor – are antinociceptive and calming in newborn infants. Different mechanisms have been proposed to account for the analgesic and quieting effects of the non-pharmacological tools we described. The effect of sucrose, sweet solutions, milk and possibly smell, seem to be mediated by the endogenous opioid system [52, 53]. The effects of pacifier and skin-to-skin contact are not blocked by naltrexone suggesting they are not mediated by the opioid system [54, 55].

Family centered approach

Most of the procedures to alleviate pain described in this paper can be implemented with parental involvement. This perspective is not only in agreement with developmental care where family members are viewed as collaborators in neonatal care, but it is also beneficial for both infants and their families. For example, when mothers spend time in skin-to-skin contact with their infants, benefits are seen in both infant and mother. Infants have better temperature and respiratory regulation, and mothers have increased breast-feeding, maternal bonding and a sense of competence [56-58]. However strategies to improve parents' involvement in daily care are still needed [59].

Pain management

Pain management is now described by researchers as a process comprising: (a) environment that is favorable to effective pain management, (b) safe preparation of the baby for the procedure, (c) pain alleviation during the procedure, and (d) restoration of the baby's sense of security after the procedure [60]. Although a vast amount of work has been done on alleviation of pain with non-invasive procedures, NICU's implementation of pain management is still insufficient [61]. Collaborative quality improvement can assist multidisciplinary neonatal intensive care unit teams in successfully implementing change [62].

Conclusion

Optimal infant pain management begins with a philosophy of care that is developmental and relationship based. Because of the potential impact of neonatal experiences on brain development and subsequent behavior but also from an ethical perspective, alleviation of pain must be an essential aspect of daily care in every NICU. Research has demonstrated the safety and effectiveness of a wide range of non-pharmacological interventions to reduce pain but implementation of pain management programs is still insufficient. Efforts should now be focused on the training of neonatal teams. These efforts offer great opportunities for nurses to contribute to scientific research to improve the care of neonates. Finally, we have to consider associating parents more closely with the care of their infants. By accepting parents as partners in the NICUs we help them to become more competent and to promote the well-being of their children.

References

1. Anand KJS, Carr DB. The neuroanatomy, neurophysiology and neurochemistry of pain, stress and analgesia in newborns and children. *Pediatr Clin North Am* 1989; 36: 795-822.

2. Anand KJS, Hickey PR. Pain and its effects in the human neonate and fetus. *N Engl J Med* 1987; 317: 1321-9.

3. Barker DP, Rutter N. Exposure to invasive procedures in neonatal intensive care unit admissions. *Arch Dis Child* 1995; 72: F47-F48.

4. Barr RG. Reflections on measuring pain in infants: dissociation in responsive systems and "honest signalling". *Arch Dis Child* 1998; 79: F152-F156.

5. Stevens B, Johnston C, Petryshen P, Taddio A. Premature infant pain profile: development and initial validation. *Clin J Pain* 1996; 12: 13-22.

6. Porter FL, Wolf CM, Miller JP. The effect of handling and immobilization on the response to acute pain in newborn infants. *Pediatrics* 1998; 102: 1383-9.

7. Als H. Toward a synactive theory of development: a promise for the assessment and support of infant individuality. *Infant Ment Health J* 1982; 3: 229-43.

8. Gottfried AW, Hodgman JE. How intensive is newborn intensive care? An environmental analysis. *Pediatrics* 1984; 74: 292-4.

9. Long JG, Phillip AGS, Lucey JF. Excessive handling as a cause of hypoxemia. *Pediatrics* 1980; 65: 203-7.

10. Murdoch DR, Darlow BA. Handling during neonatal intensive care. *Arch Dis Child* 1984; 59: 957-61.

11. Johnston CC, Stevens BJ. Experience in a neonatal intensive care unit affects pain response. *Pediatrics* 1996; 98: 925-30.

12. Johnston CC, Stevens B, Yang F, Horton L. Developmental changes in response to heelstick in preterm infants: a prospective cohort study. *Dev Med Child Neurol* 1996; 38: 438-45.

13. Als H, Lawhon G, Duffy Fh, McAnulty GB, Gibes-Grossman R, Blickman JG. Individualized developmental care for the very low-birth-weight preterm infant: medical and neurofunctional effects. *JAMA* 1994; 272: 853-8.

14. Franck LS, Lawhon G. Environmental and behavioral strategies to prevent and manage neonatal pain. *Semin Perinatol* 1998; 22: 434-43.

15. Blackburn S, Patteson D. Effects of cycled light on activity state and cardiorespiratory function in preterm infants. *J Perinat Neonatal Nurs* 1991; 4: 47-54.

16. Korner A, Thoman EB. The relative efficacy of contact and vestibular-proprioceptive stimulation on soothing neonates. *Child Dev* 1972; 2: 443-53.

17. Ferran I, Kisilevsky B, Hains SMJ. Swaddling after heel lance: Age-specific effects on behavioral recovery in preterm infants. *J Dev Behav Pediatr* 1997; 18: 222-32.

18. Campos RG. Rocking and pacifiers: two comforting interventions for heelstick pain. *Res Nurs Health* 1994; 17: 321-31.

19. Gray L, Watt L, Blass EM. Skin-to-skin contact is analgesic in healthy newborns. *Pediatrics* 2000: 105: 1-6.

20. Shah VS, Taddio A, Bennett S, Speidel BD. Neonatal pain response to heel stick *vs* venepuncture for routine blood sampling. *Arch Dis Child* 1997; 77: F143-F144.

21. Larsson BA, Tannfeldt G, Lagercrantz H, Olsson GL. Venipuncture is more effective and less painful than heel-lancing for blood tests in neonates. *Pediatrics* 1998; 101: 822-6.

22. Harpin VA, Rutter N. Making heel pricks less painful. *Arch Dis Child* 1983; 58: 226-8.

23. McIntosh N, van Veen L, Brameyer H. Alleviation of the pain of heel prick in preterm infants. *Arch Dis Child* 1994; 70: F177-F181.

24. Eriksson M, Gradin M, Schollin J. Oral glucose and venipuncture reduce blood sampling pain in newborns. *Ear Hum Dev* 1999; 55: 211-8.

25. Field T, Goldson E. Pacifying effects of non-nutritive sucking on term and preterm neonates during heelsticks. *Pediatrics* 1984; 74: 1012-5.

26. Miller H, Anderson GC. Non-nutritive sucking: effects on crying and heart rate in intubated infants requiring assisted mechanical ventilation. *Nurs Res* 1993; 42: 305-7.

27. Campos R. Soothing pain-elicited distress in infants with swaddling and pacifiers. *Child Dev* 1989; 60: 781-92.

28. Blass EM, Watt L. Suckling and sucrose-induced analgesia in human newborns. *Pain* 1999; 83: 611-23.

29. Franck L. A national survey of assessment and treatment of pain and agitation in the neonatal intensive care unit. *J Obstet Gynecol Neonatal Nurs* 1987; 16: 387-93.

30. Webster E. The use of pacifiers for non-nutritive sucking by babies in neonatal unit: a qualitative investigation into neonatal nurses' perspectives. *Journal of Neonatal Nursing* 1999; 5: 23-9.

31. Blass EM, Hoffmeyer LB. Sucrose as an analgesic for newborn infants. *Pediatrics* 1991; 87: 215-8.

32. Bucher Hu, Moser T, von Siebenthal K, Keel M, Wolf M, Duc G. Sucrose reduces pain reaction to heel lancing in preterm infant: A placebo-controlled, randomized and masked study. *Pediatr Res* 1995; 38: 332-5.

33. Haouari N, Wood C, Griffiths G, Levene M. The analgesic effect of sucrose in full term infants: a randomised controlled trial. *BMJ* 1995; 310: 1498-500.

34. Abad F, Diaz NM, Domenech E, Robayna M, Rico J. Oral sweet solutions reduces pain-related behavior in preterm infants. *Acta Paediatr* 1996; 85: 854-8.

35. Ramenghi L, Wood C, Griffeth G, Levene M. Reduction of pain response in premature infants using intraoral sucrose. *Arch Dis Child* 1996; 74: F126-F128.

36. Rushforth JA, Levene MI. Effect of sucrose on crying in response to heel stab. *Arch Dis Child* 1993; 69: 388-9.

37. Carbajal R, Lenclen R, Gajdos V, Jugie M, Paupe A. Crossover trial of analgesic efficacy of glucose and pacifier in very preterm neonates during subcutaneous injections. *Pediatrics* 2002; 110: 389-93.

38. Carbajal R, Chauvet X, Couderc S, Olivier-Martin M. Randomised trial of analgesic effects of sucrose, glucose, and pacifiers in term neonates. *BMJ* 1999; 319: 1393-7.

39. Stevens B, Taddio A, Ohlsson A, Einarson T. The efficacy of sucrose for relieving procedural pain in neonates – a systematic review and meta-analysis. *Acta Paediatr* 1997; 36: 837-42.

40. Stevens B, Yamada J, Ohlsson A. Sucrose for analgesia in newborn infants undergoing painful procedures. *Cochrane Database Syst Rev* 2001; (4): CD001069.

41. Johnston CC, Filion F, Snider L, et al. Routine sucrose analgesia during the first week of life in neonates younger than 31 weeks' postconceptional age. *Pediatrics* 2002; 110: 523-8.

42. Johnston C, Stevens B, Horton L, Stremler R. Effectiveness of oral sucrose and simulated rocking on pain response in preterm neonates. *Pain* 1997; 72: 193-9.

43. Gormally SM, Barr RG, Young SN, Alhawaf R, Wersheim L. Combined sucrose and carrying reduces newborn pain response more than sucrose or carrying alone. *Arch Pediatr Adoles Med* 1996; 150: 47.

44. Ramenghi L, Griffith G, Wood C, Levene M. Effect of non-sucrose sweet tasting solution on neonatal heel prick responses. *Arch Dis Child* 1996; 74: F129-F131.

45. Blass EM. Milk-induced hypoalgesia in human newborns. *Pediatrics* 1997; 99: 825-9.

46. Skogsdal Y, Eriksson M, Schollin J. Analgesia in newborns given oral glucose. *Acta Paediatr* 1997; 86: 217-20.

47. Gradin M, Eriksson M, Holmqvist G, Holstein A, Schollin J. Pain reduction at venipuncture in newborns: oral glucose compared with local anesthetic cream. *Pediatrics* 2002; 110: 1053-7.

48. Gray L, Miller LW, Philipp BM, Blass EM. Breast-feeding is analgesic in healthy newborns. *Pediatrics* 2002; 109: 590-3.

49. Carbajal R, Veerapen S, Couderc S, Jugie M, Ville Y. Analgesic effect of breast feeding in term neonates: randomised controlled trial. *BMJ* 2003; 326: 1-5.

50. Rattaz C, Goubet N, Bullinger A. The calming effect of a familiar odor in full-term newborns. *J Dev Behav Pediatr* 2005; 26: 86-92.

51. Goubet N, Rattaz C, Pierrat V, Bullinger A, Lequien P. Olfactory experience mediates response to pain in preterm newborns. *Dev Psychobiol* 2003; 42: 171-80.

52. Blass EM, Fitzgerald E, Kehoe P. Interactions between sucrose, pain and isolation distress. *Pharmacol Biochem Behav* 1987; 26: 483-9.

53. Blass EM, Fitzgerald E. Milk-induced analgesia and comforting in 10-day-old rats: opiod mediation. *Pharmacol Biochem Behav* 1988; 29: 9-13.

54. Blass EM, Fillion TJ, Weller A, Brunson L. Separation of opiod from nonopiod mediation of affect in neonatal rats: nonopiod mechanisms mediate maternal contact influences. *Behav Neurosci* 1990; 104: 625-36.

55. Blass EM, Shide DJ, Zaw-Mon C, Sorrentino J. Mother as shield: differential effects of contact and nursing on pain responsivity in infant rats – evidence for nonopiod mediation. *Behav Neurosci* 1995; 109: 342-53.

56. Sloan NL, Camacho LW, Rojas EP, Stern C. Kangaroo mother method: randomized controlled trial of an alternative method of care for stabilized low-birthweight infants. *Lancet* 1994; 344: 782-5.

57. Ludington-Hoe SM, Hashemi MS, Argote LA, Medellin G. Selected physiologic measures and behaviour during paternal skin contact with Colombian preterm infants. *J Dev Physiol* 1992; 18: 223-32.

58. Tessier R, Cristo M, Velez S, et al. Kangaroo mother care and the bonding hypothesis. *Pediatrics* 1998; 102: 390-1.

59. Franck LS, Spencer C. Parents visiting and participation in infant caregiving activities in a neonatal unit. *Birth* 2003; 30: 31-5.

60. Halimaa SL. Pain management in nursing procedures on premature babies. *J Adv Nurs* 2003; 42: 587-97.

61. Debillon T, Bureau V, Savagner C, Zupan-Simunek V, Carbajal R. On behalf of the French National Federation of Neonatologists. Pain management in French neonatal intensive care units. *Acta Paediatr* 2002; 91: 822-6.

62. Horbar JD, Plsek PE, Leahy K. NIC/Q 2000: Establishing habits for improvement in neonatal intensive care units. *Pediatrics* 2003; 111: e397-e410.

The Newborn Individualized Developmental Care and Assessment Program (NIDCAP)

Björn Westrup, Agneta Kleberg, Karin Stjernqvist

The mortality among infants prematurely born has dramatically decreased during the last decade in developed countries. The survival of very-low-birth-weight infants (VLBW: < 1500 g) has increased from 50% [1] to more than 85% [2] since the initiation of neonatal intensive care in the early 1970's. However, a concomitant decrease in morbidity has not yet been conclusively shown to take place. Pulmonary morbidity and neurodevelopmental outcome are the two major issues of concern [3, 4]. Employing the 1980 WHO definition of disability, follow-up studies of VLBW infants have reported the incidence to 15-25% [5, 6]. A recent meta-analysis revealed that at school age, cognitive scores of former VLBW infants are approximately 10 points lower than those of matched control children [6]. The prematurely born children also show more difficulties with attention, behaviour, visual-motor integration and language performance [7-9].

Early experience and brain development and function

Sensory input influences the structure and function of the central nervous system, as well as the behaviour of the newborn [10-13]. Infants born very prematurely receive inappropriate stimulation and care during a critical period when their brains are developing rapidly. In the germinal zone most of the neuronal multiplication and migration is complete but astrocytes are formed and subsequently migrate to upper cortical layers. Astrocytes destined for the white matter and the subcortical plate are derived from radial glial cells. Myelination begins and a naturally occurring neuronal death by apoptosis is more frequent than at any other period [14]. It has been calculated that up to 70% of neurons in the human cortex undergo apoptosis between the 28th week of gestation and term [15]. Similarly, the most active phase of synaptogenesis is initiated along with the growth of dendritic and axonal arbours. The volume of the cortical grey matter increases fourfold from 30 and 40 weeks of gestation [16]. At its maximum, as many as 40,000 new synapses are formed every second [17]. This wiring of neuronal circuits is dependent on endogenous factors as well as on sensory input and experience [17, 18].

Bearing all these extraordinary intense activities in mind, it is not surprising that the development of the brain could be disturbed by premature birth, an effect one could expect would be amplified with time if stem cell or progenitor cell proliferation were affected. A recent study of eight-year-old ex-preterm infants demonstrated with magnetic resonance imaging (MRI) technique large (12-35%) regional reductions in brain volume [19]. The strongest predictor of this reduction was not perinatal risk factors such as haemorrhage and severity of illness, or demographic factors such as gender and maternal education, but the degree of the infant's prematurity.

Nevertheless, the experience of pain and discomfort caused by treatment and caregiving procedures during the hospitalisation of VLBW infants is of great concern. Experiences of pain during the neonatal period have been linked with long-lasting accentuated stress responses [23], altered neural circuits [24], learning deficits and behavioural changes in rodents [25]. Moreover, it is difficult for VLBW infants to experience restful and undisturbed periods of sleep. During a 24-hour observation period, such infants have been reported to be handled on the average more than 200 times [20]. Three of four typical hypoxemic episodes in preterm infants have been reported to be associated with the caregiving itself [21] and increased levels of stress hormones have been observed to occur in association with routine nursing procedures [22].

Infants born very-low-birth-weight are at high risk of receiving developmentally inappropriate stimulation. They are reported to demonstrate hypersensitivity to stimuli, greater difficulties in maintaining alertness and to require more help in order to regain stability, in comparison to full-term infants [26-28]. Preterm infants are also less responsive to interaction than are full-term infants and demonstrate lower levels of signalling their availability for social bids. Since it is difficult to observe and interpret their weak signals these babies are more difficult for parents and other caregivers to predict [29].

The important role of the family in caring for VLBW infants has also been emphasised and the concept of family-centred care has been strongly advocated [30]. Minde and collaborators [29] have shown that neonatal illness may have a lasting negative effect on parent-infant interactions.

The NIDCAP

In an attempt to address these different issues, neuropsychologist Als has incorporated findings from basic science disciplines with those of developmental psychology and has formulated a new idea of care-giving. Her approach has put the focus on respect for the very tiny, but sensitive and competent, human being. She developed a theoretical framework for family-centred, developmentally supportive care, the Synactive Theory [31], which describes the infant as an organism displaying five subsystems. These are defined as the autonomic-physiological, motor, state organisational, attentional-interactive and self-regulatory subsystems. All subsystems are described as interactive, with the functional state of one system profoundly influencing the others. Thus, the stability and efficient functioning of one of these systems affects the functions of the other systems in a positive fashion. For example, helping an infant reduce his/her disorganised movements results in improved autonomic subsystem function, with improved respiration and saturation. This improvement in turn promotes the infant's ability to interact socially with the parent or caregiver. The five subsystems interact synergistically.

On the basis of this theoretical framework, Als developed the program of intervention known as the Newborn Individualized Developmental Care and Assessment Program (NIDCAP). The major approach employed in this program is through the implementation of weekly, formalised, naturalistic observations of the infant before, during and after a care-giving procedure. For example, observations might be performed around typical interactions such as feeding, changes of diaper, collection of a blood sample, or repositioning. Behavioural and physiological changes are monitored by two-minute epochs. Subsequently, the observer evaluates the infant's current ability to organise and modulate his/her subsystems and notes the infant's signals of well-being and self-regulation, as well as signals of sensitivity and stress. The infant's behaviour, described as avoidance of or approach towards stimuli, enables the observer to assess how the infant strives to cope with his/her environment and continue his/her development. These observations provide information concerning the infant's strengths and sensitivities at the point of time in question. In addition, information is obtained concerning how adequately the environment, the caregivers and family members are attuned to the current needs of the infant.

Subsequently, the observer writes a report describing in detail the behaviour of the infant during the entire observation, and develops a list of inferred developmental goals that the infant is working to achieve This report is then used to explain the behaviour of the infant in guidance of the parents and caregivers by illustrating complex interactions between the infant's different subsystems. For a trained observer this entire procedure requires 3-4 hours.

On the basis of this procedure, recommendations with respect to caregiving designed to support the individual infant's development are formulated. Such recommendations may include details on how to:

- Adjust the infant's physical environment by adjusting the levels of sound, light and activity;
- Make it easier for the infant to assume a flexed position by providing supportive bedding in the incubator, thus facilitating self-soothing/-regulatory behaviour;
- Concentrate care-giving to certain limited periods in order to allow restful sleep; and
- Help parents to understand their infant's signals, enhance their ability to recognise the infant's needs and encourage their early participation in caregiving.

Accordingly, caregivers learn to watch sensitively and note the reactions of the infant to different types of handling and care, and thus continuously make appropriate adjustments. Moreover, NIDCAP is a family-centred programme. The goal is to empower the parents by supporting them in developing such care skills and techniques, thus including the family as part of the health care team.

Currently, there are twelve training centres that provide formal training and certification of NIDCAP observers (www.nidcap.org). The training, which contains both theoretical and practical components, is quite extensive and it usually takes over a year before reliability can be achieved.

Research results

Up to this point, there have been three randomised controlled trials published on the effects on VLBW infants by a *full* implementation of NIDCAP [32-34]. In the recent meta-analysis by Jacobs and collaborators, they report separately on these three RCTs and indicate that these studies demonstrate positive short-term effects among the NIDCAP infants in regards to pulmonary morbidity. The studies document a mean difference in mechanical ventilation of 25.7 days (95% CI: 7.5; 43.9) in favour of the intervention as well as a reduction of supplementary oxygen by 41.1 days (16.8; 65.3) [35]. A Cochrane Review [36] also reported a relative risk for the NIDCAP infants of moderate-severe pulmonary radiographic findings of 0.34 (95% CI: 0.15; 0.81). In addition, from our own calculations, the relative risk of intraventricular haemorrhages of grade III or more for the NIDCAP infants is 0.51 (95% CI: 0.23; 1.1). The positive impact on short-term medical outcome has been confirmed by two recent reports – one from a larger [37] and the other from a multi-centre RCT [38].

Jacobs and co-workers report a mean difference in the mental developmental index assessed by the Bayley Scales of Infant Development at 9-12 months of age of + 16.6 (95% CI: 9.3; 23.8) in favour of the NIDCAP infants [35]. In this meta-analysis, the longest follow-up period of a single study was two years of corrected age [39]. The mental indices in this study were in favour of the NIDCAP group but the difference was not statistically significant. However, this study was not dimensioned for the follow-up phase of the study and, thus the power the analysis was low. Furthermore, one third of the original sample was lost at the time of the reported assessment.

A recent report [40] from a five year follow up of the Swedish randomised control trial (RCT) demonstrated a significant impact on the NIDCAP group only in the behavioural aspect of development. The Odds Ratio (OR) for surviving without abnormal behaviour was 19.9 (95% CI: 1.1- > 100). The corresponding OR for survival without mental retardation was 3.5 (0.7- > 100) and without overall disability 14.7 (0.8- > 100). There were no subjects lost in this follow-up but, for the same reason as in the previous study, the power was low.

In two RCTs, assessment of neurophysiological functions was performed with evoked potentials and quantitative topographic mapping of electroencephalograms (brain electrical area mapping; BEAM) [32, 41]. Both of these studies revealed significant differences in favour of NIDCAP intervention. Interestingly, in the study on the more mature, low-risk infants, the largest differences were observed in the frontal lobe area, where neuronal organisation occurs relatively late [41]. Using quantitative 3D-magnetic resonance imaging techniques and diffusion tensor imaging, the same investigators recently presented preliminary data that indicated beneficial changes in tissue distribution as well as in micro structural development of white matter in NIDCAP infants compared with control group infants at term age [42].

The complexity of developmentally supportive care and its demand for comprehensive training has caused some concern about its cost-effectiveness [36]. However, several groups have reported that NIDCAP actually reduces costs by $4,000-120,000 per infant depending on his/her birthweight and initial illness [32, 33, 43]. Concerns have also been expressed that the implementation of this program would require extra nursing time. However, according to three different European investigations NIDCAP increases the competence of both staff members and parents [46-48]. Caregiving is specifically adjusted to the current medical and developmental status of the infant. It might be speculated that the caregivers become more skilled and detect changes in the infant's status at an earlier stage. This might, in turn, lead to prompt intervention and prevention of further deterioration. Thus, the infants become more physiologically stable and actually require less nursing time, which is in line with the findings of others [49, 50].

In addition, studies on effects of NIDCAP components in *specific* care-giving situations have recently been reported. Sizun and co-workers demonstrated decreased pain response and fewer hypoxic events during a routine nursing procedure in medically stable preterm infants [44]. A preliminary report from the same group of investigators also indicates increased duration of sleep in infants receiving developmental care [45].

Discussion

Intervention such as the NIDCAP approach, which includes individualised, baby and family sensitive intervention is attractive from an ethical point of view [51]. The basis of family-centred developmentally supportive care is based on a recognition that the newborn infant is a human being in his/her own right and encourage caregivers to be guided by the current needs of the individual infant and its family. However, published studies on the effects of NIDCAP have been relatively few, with small numbers and so far with relatively short follow-up periods. The methodology of these studies has been questioned [35, 36]. Due to the complexity of the intervention, evaluation of NIDCAP is complicated in comparison to studies involving, for example, different drug treatments or modes of ventilation. It is difficult to achieve an optimal experimental design for studies with a high degree of complexity. Additionally, there is no gold standard for nursing care, making the definition of the control group variable. The intervention cannot be applied in a blinded fashion. The experiments may include several individual approaches, which result in confounding factors, and a single procedure may not be analysed separately.

The duration of integrated care approaches such as NIDCAP for more vulnerable infants lasts for months, resulting in the risk of spill over effects on the control group. Moreover, parents share experiences with each other and actively seek knowledge designed to improve the treatment of their infant, further contributing to challenges in implementing well designed and controlled studies.

Most studies of individual interventions labelled as developmental care include small numbers of generally healthy preterm newborns and thus, the results are not readily generalisable for infants with acute illness and/or extreme prematurity as is inherent in the NIDCAP approach. An early Swedish study has indicated that environmental changes in the neonatal unit are not in themselves sufficient to explain the improvement observed in studies using the NIDCAP approach [46]. During periods without formal NIDCAP observations, there was an obvious decline in the quality of care. Thus, to achieve consistent improvement in outcomes, regular observations appear to be essential, although to what extent remains to be determined.

It is important to emphasise that not all personnel are suited to become NIDCAP observers. It requires a good deal of sensitivity to interpret the subtle signs of a premature infant and a great deal of psychological skill to interact with the staff and parents in such a manner that they feel supported and not criticised. Implementation of developmental care in the hands of an unskilled person involves a potential risk of over-emphasising the "protection" of the infant, that is, to forget the individualised portion of the program. NIDCAP ought not be implemented unreflectively. For example, completely covering of the incubator of a not-yet-stabilised infant, thereby preventing its necessary surveillance; building containment for the infant which is too rigid; and over-protecting a stable, competent baby from visual, auditory and social input, thus preventing development of it's the ability to self-regulate and interact socially. Instead, intervention should be designed from the viewpoint of each individual infant. Determining what is appropriate for the particular infant at the particular time, considering all factors, including the infant's medical status is at the heart of the individualised NIDCAP approach.

Conclusion

The theoretical framework behind family-centred developmentally supportive care/NIDCAP is endorsed by research from several scientific fields such as neuroscience, developmental and family psychology, medicine and nursing. However, the introduction of NIDCAP is not a trivial process, Implementation of the NIDCAP approach involves a considerable investment at all levels of the organisation. NIDCAP requires some physical changes in the NICU, as well as substantial educational efforts and changes in the practice of care. The findings of our own investigations on the effects of NIDCAP have been encouraging and in line with the results of previous studies. NIDCAP has been very well received by nursing staff, neonatologists and parents [46-48, 52]. It is attractive from an ethical perspective, as well. It appears reasonable to recommend nurseries to acquire the expertise to implement NIDCAP in order to be able to engage in new and much warranted investigations of developmentally supportive care, in different cultural contexts and with diversified and, if possible, larger, randomised multi-centre trials.

References

1. Stewart AL, Reynolds EO, Lipscomb AP. Outcome for infants of very low birthweight: Survey of world literature. *Lancet* 1981; 1: 1038-40.

2. Horbar JD, Badger GJ, Lewit EM, Rogowski J, Shiono PH. Hospital and patient characteristics associated with variation in 28-day mortality rates for very low birth weight infants. Vermont Oxford Network. *Pediatrics* 1997; 99: 149-56.

3. Vaucher YE. Bronchopulmonary dysplasia: an enduring challenge. *Pediatr Rev* 2002; 23: 349-58.

4. Bregman J. Developmental outcome in very low birthweight infants. Current status and future trends. *Pediatr Clin North Am* 1998; 45: 673-90.

5. Bylund B, Cervin T, Finnstrom O, *et al*. Morbidity and neurological function of very low birthweight infants from the newborn period to 4 years of age. A prospective study from the south-east region of Sweden. *Acta Paediatr* 1998; 87: 758-63.

6. Bhutta AT, Cleves MA, Casey PH, Cradock MM Anand KJS. Cognitive and behavioural outcomes of school-aged children who were born preterm: a meta-analysis. *JAMA* 2002; 288: 728-37.

7. Hack M, Fanaroff AA. Outcomes of children of extremely low birthweight and gestational age in the 1990's. *Early Hum Dev* 1999; 53: 193-218.

8. Stjernqvist K, Svenningsen NW. Ten-year follow-up of children born before 29 gestational weeks: health, cognitive development, behaviour and school achievement. *Acta Paediatr* 1999; 88: 557-62.

9. Wolke D, Meyer R. Cognitive status, language attainment, and prereading skills of 6-year-old very preterm children and their peers: the Bavarian Longitudinal Study. *Dev Med Child Neurol* 1999; 4: 94-109.

10. Wiesel TN, Hubel DH. Comparison of the effects of unilateral and bilateral eye closure on cortical unit responses in kittens. *J Neurophysiol* 1965; 28: 1029-40.

11. Philbin MK, Ballweg DD, Gray L. The effect of an intensive care unit sound environment on the development of habituation in healthy avian neonates. *Dev Psychobiol* 1994; 27: 11-21.

12. Modney BK, Hatton GI. Maternal behaviors: evidence that they feed back to alter brain morphology and function. *Acta Paediatrica suppl.* 1994; 397: 29-32.

13. Rosenblum LA, Andrews MW. Influences of environmental demand on maternal behavior and infant development. *Acta Paediatrica suppl.* 1994; 397: 57-63.

14. Evrard P, Marret S, Gressens P. Environmental and genetic determinants of neural migration and postmigratory survival. *Acta Paediatrica suppl.* 1997; 422: 20-6.

15. Rabinowicz T, de Courten-Myers GM, Petetot JM, Xi G, de los Reyes E. Human cortex development: estimates of neuronal numbers indicate major loss late during gestation. *J Neuropathol Exp Neurol* 1996; 55: 320-8.

16. Huppi PS, Warfield S, Kikinis R, *et al*. Quantitative magnetic resonance imaging of brain development in premature and mature newborns. *Ann Neurol* 1998; 43: 224-35.

17. Bourgeois JP. Synaptogenesis, heterochrony and epigenesis in the mammalian neocortex. *Acta Paediatrica suppl.* 1997; 422: 27-33.

18. Penn AA, Shatz CJ. Brain waves and brain wiring: the role of endogenous and sensory-driven neural activity in development. *Ped Res* 1999; 45: 447-58.

19. Peterson BS, Vohr B, Staib LH, *et al*. Regional brain volume abnormalities and long-term cognitive outcome in preterm infants. *JAMA* 2000; 284: 1939-47.

20. Murdock D. Handling during neonatal intensive care. *Arch Dis Child* 1984; 59: 957-61.

21. Long JG, Lucey JF, Philip AG. Noise and hypoxemia in the intensive care nursery. *Pediatrics* 1980; 65: 143-5.

22. Lagercrantz H, Nilsson E, Redham I, Hjelmdahl P. Plasma catecholamines following nursing procedures in a neonatal ward. *Early Hum Dev* 1986; 14: 61-5.

23. Liu D, Caldji C, Sharma S, Plotsky PM, Meaney MJ. Influence of neonatal rearing conditions on stress-induced adrenocorticotropin responses and norepinepherine release in the hypothalamic paraventricular nucleus. *J Neuroendocrinol* 2000; 12: 5-12.

24. Ruda MA, Ling QD, Hohmann AG, Peng YB, Tachibana T. Altered nociceptive neuronal circuits after neonatal peripheral inflammation. *Science* 2000; 289: 628-31.

25. Anand KJ, Coskun V, Thrivikraman KV, Nemeroff CB, Plotsky PM. Long-term behavioral effects of repetitive pain in neonatal rat pups. *Physiol Behav* 1999; 66: 627-37.

26. Als H, McAnulty GB. Behavioral differences between preterm and full-term newborns as measured with the APIB system scores: I. *Infant Behavior and Development* 1988; 11: 305-18.

27. Stjernqvist K, Svenningsen NW. Neurobehavioral development at term of extremely low-birthweight infants (less than 901g). *Dev Med Child Neurol* 1990; 32: 679-88.

28. Eckerman CO, Oehler JM, Medvin MB, Hannan TE. Premature newborns as social partners before term age. *Infant Behavior and Development* 1994; 17: 55-70.

29. Minde K, Whitelaw A, Brown J, Fitzhardinge P. Effect of neonatal complications in premature infants on early parent-infant interactions. *Dev Med Child Neurol* 1983; 25: 763-77.

30. Harrison H. The principles for family-centered neonatal care [see comments]. *Pediatrics* 1993; 92: 643-50.

31. Als H, Lawhon G, Brown E, et al. Individualized behavioural and environmental care for the very low birth weight preterm infant at high risk for bronchopulmonary dysplasia: Neonatal intensive care unit and developmental outcome. *Pediatrics* 1986; 78: 1123-32.

32. Als H, Lawhon G, Duffy FH, McAnulty GB, Gibes-Grossman R, Blickman JG. Individualized developmental care for the very low-birth-weight preterm infant. Medical and neurofunctional effects. *JAMA* 1994; 272: 853-8.

33. Fleisher BE, VandenBerg K, Constantinou J, et al. Individualized developmental care for very low birthweight premature infants improves medical and neurodevelopmental outcome in the neonatal intensive care unit. *Clin Pediatr* 1995; 34: 523-9.

34. Westrup B, Kleberg A, von Eichwald K, Stjernqvist K, Lagercrantz H. A randomised controlled trial to evaluate the effects of NIDCAP (Newborn Individualized Developmental Care and Assessment Program) in a Swedish setting. *Pediatrics* 2000; 105: 66-72.

35. Jacobs SE, Sokol J, Ohlsson A. The Newborn Individualized Developmental Care and Assessment Program is not supported by meta-analyses of the data. *J Pediatr* 2002; 140: 699-706.

36. Symington A, Pinelli J. Developmental care for promoting development and preventing morbidity in preterm infants. *Cochrane Database Syst Rev* 2003; (4): CD001814.

37. Tyebkhan JM, Peters KL, Cote JJ, McPherson CA, Hendson L. The impact of developmental care in the NICU: The Edmonton Randomized Controlled Trial of NIDCAP. *Pediatr Res* 2004; 55: 505A.

38. Als H, Gilkerson L, Duffy FH, et al. A three-center, randomized, controlled trial of individualized developmental care for very low birth weight preterm infants: medical, neurodevelopmental, parenting, and caregiving effects. *J Dev Behav Pediatr* 2003; 24: 399-408.

39. Ariagno RL. Developmental care does not alter sleep and development in premature infants. *Pediatrics* 1997; 100 (6): E9.

40. Westrup B, Böhm B, Lagercrantz H, Stjernqvist K. Preschool outcome in children born very preterm and cared according to NIDCAP. *Acta Paediatr* 2004; 93: 498-507.

41. Buehler DM, Als H, Duffy FH, McAnulty GB, Liederman J. Effectiveness of individualized developmental care for low-risk preterm infants: Behavioural and electrophysiologic evidence. *Pediatrics* 1995; 96: 923-32.

42. Als H, Duffy FH, McAnulty GB, et al. Early experience alters brain function and structure. *Pediatrics* 2004; 113: 846-57.

43. Petryshen P, Stevens B, Hawkins J, Stewart M. Comparing nursing costs for preterm infants receiving conventional *vs.* developmental care. *Nurs Econ* 1997; 15: 138-45 150.

44. Sizun J, Ansquer H, Browne J, Tordjman S, Morin JF. Developmental care decreases physiologic and behavioural pain expression in preterm neonates. *J Pain* 2002; 3: 446-50.

45. Bertelle V, Mabin D, Curzi L, Adrien J, Sizun J. Sleep of preterm neonates under developmental care or regular environmental conditions. *Early Hum Dev* 2005; 81: 595-600.

46. Westrup B, Kleberg A, Wallin L, Lagercrantz H, Wikblad K, Stjernqvist K. Evaluation of the Newborn Individualized Developmental Care and Assessment Program (NIDCAP) in a Swedish setting. *Prenat Neonat Med* 1997; 2: 366-75.

47. Mambrini C, Dobrzynski M, Ratynski N, Sizun J, de Parscau L. Implantation des soins de développement et comportement du personnel soignant. *Arch Pédiatr* 2002; 9 S: 104-6.

48. Rémont C, Schoutteten C, Hennequin Y, Vermeylen D, Pardou A. *Satisfaction of the carers during NIDCAP program implementation*. International Conference on Infant Development in Neonatal Intensive Care. London: 2003: 38.

49. Stevens B, Petryshen P, Hawkins J, Smith B, Taylor P. Developmental versus conventional care: A comparison of clinical outcomes for very low birth weight infants. *Can J Nurs Res* 1996; 28: 97-113.

50. Brown LD, Heermann JA. The effect of developmental care on preterm infant outcome. *Appl Nurs Res* 1997; 10: 190-97.

51. Kennell JH. The Humane Neonatal Care Initiative. *Acta Paediatr* 1999; 88: 367-70.

52. Westrup B, Stjernqvist K, Kleberg A, Hellstrom-Westas L, Lagercrantz H. Neonatal individualized care in practice: a Swedish experience. *Semin Neonatol* 2002; 7: 447-57.

Implementing developmental care: Considerations for staff

Inga Warren, Marina Cuttini

The creation of an environment that minimises stress while providing developmentally appropriate experience for the infant and family is the goal of developmental care. The onus on staff is to constantly keep the needs of the baby and family in mind; to do this it is necessary to also keep the needs of staff in mind.

Where developmental care in the NIDCAP (Newborn Individualised Developmental Care and Assessment Program) model has been successfully implemented, staff generally has a positive attitud towards the benefits for the baby [1, 2]. The area most likely to cause concern is the impact on working conditions. This article will explore some of the physical attributes of the nursery environment, as well as the impact of events, and organisational structures.

The physical environment of the NICU

Lighting

Traditionally nurseries have been brightly lit on the grounds that this is necessary to observe the baby and to carry out demanding tasks; in addition lighting has been perceived as harmless to babies. Developmental care takes the view that low lighting is beneficial for preterm infants, with recommendations for either continuously dimmed light, or cycles of near darkness at night with moderate daytime lighting. The 200 lux recommended in the daytime for babies [3] is considerably lower than the 2500 lux that has been recommended for staff carrying out procedures [4]. Staff may raise concerns about being able to observe babies who are shaded with incubator covers although Brandon [5] found that this could be managed safely if babies were regularly checked with the use of pen torches.

Unrelenting bright lighting can be detrimental to staff, causing fatigue, headaches and jitteriness [6]. On the other hand staff working night shifts may find it difficult to adjust their circadian rhythms without exposure to bright light during these shifts [7, 8]. Ideally nursery design should ensure that appropriate spotlighting is available for specific tasks, and that areas with daylight or good substitutes are provided for desktop tasks and rest breaks.

Noise

Low activity and noise levels are generally seen as beneficial in the work place and are promoted by developmental care. Working in a noisy environment can cause physiological stress, fatigue, irritability and mood disturbance [9]. In order to protect infant sleep and stability, and for the comfort of staff and parents, it is recommended that background noise in the nursery should not exceed an average of 50 dB with peaks not more than 70 dB [10]. Mean noise levels over 70 dB, and peaks of over 90 db have been recorded in some nurseries [11, 12]. Isolated noises that are loud enough to result in discomfort for the baby can be caused by simple activities such as putting a bottle down on the top of an incubator [13], or closing the door sharply. Some NICU workers may find it difficult to adapt their temperament to working in and creating quieter conditions.

Perceptions of noise are subjective but some sounds are generally more irritating than others; in particular the repetitive high-pitched sounds of unchecked monitor and pump alarms may be perceived to be noxious. Noise in the workplace is responsible for errors [14] and also changes the nature of communications [9]. In a noisy environment people tend to adopt a louder, more staccato style of speech that may appear abrupt or aggressive. Controlling noise in the nursery is likely to be beneficial to babies, parents, and staff alike with better staff performance and more positive styles of interaction. However, managing noise through changing staff behaviour can be difficult to sustain and, as with lighting, design features can make a significant difference.

Space

Before family centred care became a byword the idea that babies need less space than children and adults because they are small dictated nursery design. In many NICUs staff has to work in very cramped conditions, far from the recommended minimum of 14 square metres per bed space with a distance of 8 ft between cots [10]. These conditions make it difficult to protect babies and families from environmental stressors, to implement kangaroo mother care, and breast feeding. Recently there has been a move towards nursery design with single rooms for babies and their families. While this has great benefits for the privacy and involvement of the family and for organising the environment to suit individual infants, staff may feel isolated and miss the camaraderie of working together in larger groups unless space is provided for communal work and relaxation areas away from the baby's bed. Managers may fear that higher staffing levels will be needed in order to monitor babies safely but in practice these fears are unfounded if the design facilitates observation and if appropriate communications systems are in place [15].

Events in the nursery

Timing

Developmental care is baby-led, *i.e.* adjusted to suit the baby's rhythms, stability and state. This can be difficult for staff used to working by the clock, fitting care around ward routines. Routines typically reduce effort and novices may depend on them as coping strategies while mastering skills. Outside forces, such as laboratory and technician availability, are additional constraints on planning the baby's day in a personal way. Negotiation and innovation may be needed to adjust incompatible timetables of team members and support services, taking into account infant and family needs.

Concerns have been expressed that developmental care will take more time. While cares may take longer the result is likely to be a more organised, self-regulated, stable baby who is actually less demanding. Making difficult procedures easier for the baby can facilitate examinations and make treatment more effective. NIDCAP studies show a trend towards reduced need for some aspects of intensive care [16, 17] thus potentially reducing the burden on staff.

Parents' role and interactions with staff

Parents' free visiting in the NICU and involvement in the care of their babies represents a key element of developmental care. In theory, this is not a new concept. As early as 1907, Pierre Budin supported the role of mothers in the care of hospitalised preterm babies [18]. Yet subsequently the emergence of neonatology as a recognized medical speciality, focussing on technological progress and fear of infections, led to a policy of almost total exclusion of parents from the NICUs [19].

It was only in the seventies that concerns about the ill effects of mother-infant separation started to be raised [20-22]. More recently, research on the maturation of the human brain [23-25] and the increased understanding of the capabilities of the neonate have clarified the importance of the early relationships of the babies with their caregivers to counteract the distress of hospitalisation, and improve chances for optimal development. Maternal presence increases breast-feeding rates [26] and offers opportunities for Kangaroo Care, resulting in benefits on infant growth and stabilization. Additionally, baby's holding by parents is an effective type of non-pharmacological pain control during invasive medical procedures.

Parent presence with their baby is beneficial not only for the baby, but also for the parents themselves. Negative reactions to premature birth, such as anxiety, depression, fear and helplessness [27] are reduced by the contact with their baby. Active involvement in their infant's care decreases the parents' feelings of impotence and improves their sense of control, as well as actual competence. Increased satisfaction with medical care appears to be an added benefit. Being able to assist during medical procedures (by touching, talking to, and maintaining eye contact with their baby), seems to be more acceptable to parents than most physicians believe, and decreases procedure-related parental anxiety [28, 29]. Parents however should always have the choice of opting out [30].

Today, many NICUs strive to maintain and encourage close parent-child relationships, but the situation varies in different countries. An international study showed that in some European countries many NICUs still restrict family visiting *(figure 1)*. Grandparents appear even less tolerated in NICUs than siblings [31]. Such restrictive policies toward family visiting appear to extend to parents' presence during doctors' rounds and routine medical procedures, and also to access to information regarding their child [31]. To some extent, the international differences correspond to a North-South contrast: units from Northern countries (Great Britain and Sweden) appear more receptive to parental involvement than the Southern Mediterranean ones (Italy and Spain), while Germany, France and the Netherlands occupy an intermediate position.

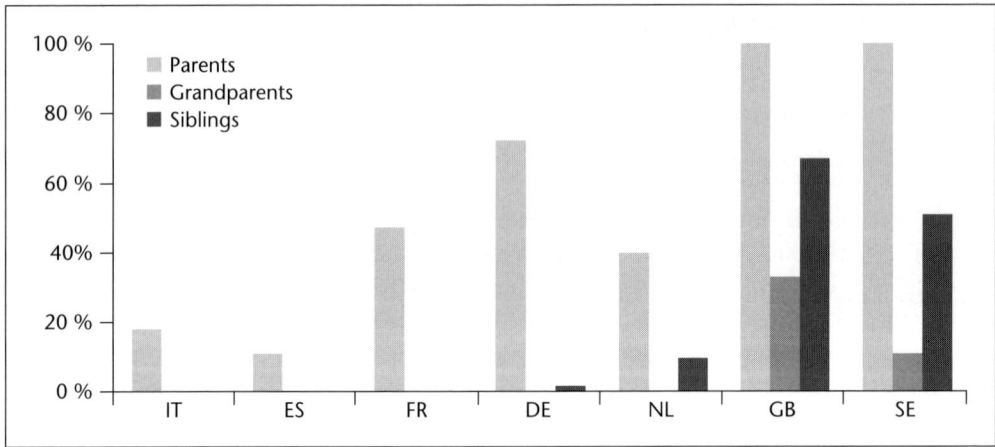

Figure 1. Proportion of Units allowing unrestricted family visiting by country.
Data are derived from Cuttini *et al. Arch Dis Child, Fetal Neonatal Ed* 1999; 81: F84-F91.

Fear of parents being too critical or "irrational", disturbance of unit routines, and increased workload are reported by staff as primary obstacles to the implementation of a more open attitude toward parents in NICUs. Such negative attitudes however are more prevalent among the staff of the units still restricting visiting *(table I)*. When the staff is already accustomed to the parents' presence, a less worried attitud is reported [32]. These findings suggest that changes of NICU policy, although initially may be perceived as threatening and meet staff opposition, eventually become more acceptable with time as staff get familiar with them and start to appreciate the positive aspects of parents' presence.

Table I. Comparison of staff and mothers' attitudes and experiences according to Unit policy (open *versus* restricted).

	Open policy Units		Restricted policy Units		P value §
	n.	(%)	n.	(%)	
STAFF VIEWS					
Parental visiting should be:					
– Unlimited	94	(89.5)	8	(13.3)	***
– Restricted to certain hours	11	(10.5)	52	(86.7)	
– Not allowed	0	/	0	/	
Parental visiting:					
– Is beneficial to infants' health	78	(74.3)	29	(48.3)	***
– Can shorten hospital stay	73	(70.2)	29	(48.3)	**
– Interferes with unit's routines	20	(19.6)	37	(63.8)	***
– Valuable for parents but stressful for staff	41	(39.8)	40	(66.7)	**
– Useful for staff	66	(62.9)	22	(38.6)	**
MOTHERS' EXPERIENCE					
Frequency of visiting: every day	39	(81.3)	25	(78.1)	NS
Average time spent with baby per visit: Median in minutes (range)	110	(30-360)	42	(10-90)	
Would like to visit more	41	(85.4)	29	(90.6)	NS
Reasons for not visiting more:					
– Not allowed	0	/	18	(62.1)	***
– Distance/costs	16	(38.1)	7	(24.1)	
– Family/health	19	(45.2)	5	(16.1)	
Breastfeeding at four weeks	28	(58.3)	5	(16.1)	***

§: *: p < 0.05; **: p < 0.01; ***: p < 0.001.
Reproduced with permission from Cuttini *et al*. Arch Dis Child, Fetal Neonatal Ed 2000; 82 (2): F172.

Yet, it should be recognized that close and continuous interactions with parents may at times become stressful for the staff, particularly for nurses. Ways of coping with difficult family members and situations should be identified within the unit. Opportunities for discussion with the other staff, and when necessary professional psychological support, can alleviate some of the stresses of interacting with parents on a daily basis.

When asked their opinion, parents consistently state that they want to be able to spend time with their baby at their own pace, and without unnecessary limitations; to receive early, direct and detailed information in a comprehensible and sympathetic manner, and to be together when given "bad news" [33]. Time to listen to the parents' concerns and understand their expectations may be hard to find in a busy unit, but is definitely crucial [34, 35]. Answering honestly the parents' questions is important yet often difficult. To minimize the chances of providing contradictory information, each baby should have his/her doctor acting as main reference person for communicating with parents. Information about parents' presence, interactions with their baby and communication with staff should be routinely included in the medical records and nurses' notes, and discussed during clinical rounds along with the other clinical matters. Supporting parents and promoting optimal interactions between them and their babies is as important to the patients' well-being as is the quality of provided medical care.

Organisation

Adopting developmental care is a gradual process. It can be challenging for staff at the early stages of integrating developmental care into their practice to work alongside those that are more advanced, and vice versa. Parents tend to perceive developmental care as good for their baby and may wonder about lack of consistency in the approach of different staff members. For developmental care to be truly effective it needs to be part of the unit culture, not an individual option; managers must be involved and the whole team must understand and subscribe to a developmental care philosophy. NIDCAP training centres ask applicants to obtain the endorsement of managers and clinical leaders before beginning training; without this preparation, individual efforts are hard to sustain and difficult to transmit to the rest of the team. In one unit this problem was addressed through a consultation process in which all staff were invited to contribute to a Charter for Developmental Care [36]. While not expecting perfection, the resulting consensus statement expresses the intention to provide a developmentally and family centred environment that is also supportive of staff. The written statement is given to all applicants for work on the unit so that they understand the expectation to contribute, as best as they can, to developmental care from the start of their appointment.

NICUs tend to be closed systems with the characteristics of emergency services, *i.e.* that team members need to know each other well, and to be able to depend on each other. Staffing structures are often hierarchical and skill requirements highly specific [37]. These qualities can create impermeable boundaries for personnel on the fringes of the team, such as therapists, who need to undergo a period of preparation, learning and supervised practice. They also need to demonstrate a stable commitment to the team in order for their contribution to the service to be valued.

Developmental care requires skills that come more naturally to some than to others. An understanding of the concepts and research as well as practice in observing and interpreting infant behaviour are essential. As yet education and training opportunities are frustratingly scarce in Europe and educational strategies are urgently needed for the future.

Staff support

In her book *Sent before my Time*, Margaret Cohen [38] talks about the need to "keep the baby in mind", and about the baby being at the centre of a complex web of relevant issues. This is the essence of developmental care. Observing babies is not an easy task, and it is often even a painful one. How do doctors and nurses keep the baby in mind when there are so many things going on in the NICU, when they see babies enduring painful procedures and separation from their parents? Cohen stresses the importance of opportunities for doctors and nurses to reflect on their experience and to vent feelings if they are able to do this work of keeping the baby in mind. To do developmental care on one's own is hardly possible; the implication for staff is the need for skilled support, without which it is hard to keep going.

References

1. Sell E. *Views of physicians/NNPs in USA NIDCAP training centers on NIDCAP and Philosophy of Family Centred care.* NIDCAP Trainers Meeting, McCall, Idaho, 1997.

2. Westrup B, Stjernqvist K, Kleberg A, Hellstrom-Westas L, Lagercrantz H. Neonatal individualized care in practice: a Swedish experience. *Semin Neonatol.* 2002; 7: 447-57.

3. Rivkees SA, Haiping H. Developing circadian rhythmicity, *Semin Perinatol* 2000; 24: 232-42.

4. White R. Recommended standards for newborn ICU design. Committee to establish recommended standards for newborn NICU design. *J Perinatol* 1999; 19: S1-S12.

5. Brandon D, Holditch-Davis D, Belya M. Preterm infants born at less than 31 weeks gestation have improved growth in cycled light compared with continuous near darkness, *J Pediatr* 2002; 140: 192-9.

6. Terman M, Terman JS. Bright light therapy: side effects and benefits across the symptom spectrum. *J Clin Psychiatry* 1999; 29: 124-7.

7. Czeisler CA, Johnson MP, Duffy JF, Brown EN, Ronda JM, Kronauer RE. Exposure to bright light and darkness to treat physiologic maladaptation to night work. *N Engl J Med* 1990; 322: 1253-9.

8. Figueiro M, Rea M, Boyce P, White R, Kolberg K. The effect of bright light on day night shift nurses, performance and well-being in the NICU. *Neonatal Intensive Care* 2001; 14: 29-32i.

9. Philbin KA, Martin PA. The acoustic environment of hospital nurseries. NICU sound environment and the potential problems for caregivers. *J Perinatol* 2000; 20: S94-S99.

10. White R. *Recommended Standards for Newborn ICU Design.* Report of the Consensus Committee to Establish Recommended Standards for Newborn ICU Design. http://www.nd.edu-kkolberg/frmain.htm 2003.

11. Philbin MK. The full-term and premature newborn. The influence of auditory experience on the behaviour of preterm newborns. *J Perinatol* 2000; 20: S77-S87.

12. Robertson A, Cooper-Peel C, Vos P. Peak noise distribution in the neonatal intensive care nursery. *J Perinatol* 1998; 18: 361-4.

13. Thomas KA. How the NICU environment sounds to a preterm infant. *Am J Matern Child Nurs* 1989; 14: 249-51.

14. Kjellberg A. Subjective, behavioural and psychophysiological effects of noise. *Scand J Work Environ Health* 1990; 16 (suppl. 1): 29-38.

15. Brown P, Taquino LT. Designing and delivering neonatal care in single rooms. *J Perinat Neonatal Nurs* 2001; 15: 68-83.

16. Stevens B, Petryshen P, Hawkins J, Stewart M. Developmental *vs.* conventional care: a comparison of clinical outcomes for very low birth weight infants. *Can J Nurs Res* 1996; 28: 97-113.

17. Westrup B, Kleberg A, von Eichwald K, Stjernqvist K, Lagercrantz H. A randomised controlled trial to evaluate the effects of Newborn Individualised Developmental Care and Assessment Programme in a Swedish setting. *Pediatrics* 2000; 105: 66-72.

18. Budin P. *The nursing*. London: Caxton Publishing, 1907.

19. Leigh Davis RM, Mohay H, Edwards H. Mothers' involvement in caring for their premature infants: an historical overview. *J Adv Nursing* 2003; 42: 578-86.

20. Barnett C, Leiderman P, Grobstein R, Klaus M. Neonatal separation: the maternal side of interactional deprivation. *Pediatrics* 1970; 45: 197-205.

21. Bowlby J. *Attachment. Vol.1.* Harmondsworth: Penguin, 1971.

22. Klaus MH, Kennel JH. *Maternal-infant bonding*. St Louis: Mosby, 1976.

23. Penn AA, Shatz CJ. Brain waves and brain wiring: the role of endogenous and sensory-driven neural activity in development. *Pediatr Res* 1999; 45: 447-58.

24. Committee on integrating the science of early childhood development. The developing brain. In: Shonkoff JP, Phillips DA, eds. From neurons to neighborhoods: the science of early childhood development. *National Academy Press* 2000: 182-218.

25. Lagercrantz H, Ringstedt T. Organization of the neuronal circuits in the central nervous system during development. *Acta Paediatr* 2001; 90: 707-15.

26. Cuttini M, Crisma M, Chiandotto V, Della Barba B, Frigieri G, Zanini R. Breastfeeding and Neonatal Intensive Care Unit policies. *Int J Epidemiol* 1997; 26: 1401-2.

27. Doering LV, Moser DK, Dracup K. Correlates of anxiety, hostility, depression and psychosocial adjustment in parents of NICU infants. *Neonatal Netw* 2000; 19: 15-23.

28. Bauchner H, Vinci R, Bak S, Pearson C, Corwin MJ. Parents and procedures: a randomized controlled trial. *Pediatrics* 1996; 98: 861-7.

29. Powers KS, Rubenstein JS. Family presence during invasive procedures in the pediatric intensive care unit: a prospective study. *Arch Pediatr Adolesc Med* 1999; 153: 955-8.

30. Cescutti-Butler L, Galvin K. Parents' perceptions of staff competency in a neonatal intensive care unit. *J Clin Nurs* 2003; 12: 752-61.

31. Cuttini M, Rebagliato M, Bortoli P, et al. Parental Visiting, Communication and Participation in Ethical Decisions: A Comparison of Neonatal Unit Policies in Europe. *Arch Dis Child Fetal Neonatal Ed* 1999; 81: F84-F91.

32. Cuttini M, Chiandotto V, Dalla Barba B, Cavazzutti Gb, Reid M. Visiting Policies In Neonatal Intensive Care Units: Staff And Parents' Views. *Arch Dis Child, Fetal Neonatal Ed* 2000; 82: F172.

33. Harrison H. The Principles For Family-Centered Neonatal Care. *Pediatrics* 1993; 92: 643-9.

34. Ward K. Perceived needs of parents of critically ill infants in a neonatal intensive care unit (nicu). *Pediatr Nurs* 2001; 27: 281-6.

35. Loo KK, Espinosa M, Tyles R, Howard J. Using knowledge to cope with stress in the nicu: how parents integrate learning to read the physiologic and behavioural cues of the infant. *Neonatal Netw* 2003; 22: 31-7.

36. Warren I. *Guidelines for Infant Development in the Newborn Nursery*. London: The Winnicott Foundation, 2001.

37. Keilhofner G. *A Model of Human Occupation: Theory and Application*. Baltimore: Williams and Wilkins, 1985.

38. Cohen M. *Sent Before My Time*. London: Karnac Books, 2003.

Clinical evaluation of development for research

Claudine Amiel-Tison, Julie Gosselin

It is reasonable to assume that adverse environmental factors in the immediate postnatal period will have unfavourable effects on brain organization in the very low birth weight (VLBW) infant. Is it possible to evaluate the contribution of those factors on developmental sequelae in this high-risk group of infants? This chapter focuses on the current methodological principles of follow-up studies and proposes a plausible strategy to measure the potential effects of developmental care on long-term outcome with a new look at the neurological exam. The main pitfalls related to a valid appreciation of efficacy as well as the qualitative value of developmental care are also discussed.

Methodological principles of follow-up studies

Even though significant methodological differences exist among long-term outcome studies of high risk neonates, general principles may be identified.

Neurological assessment at 40 weeks corrected

Many types of neurological assessments of the newborn infant have been described in the last decades. A recent review compares the definitions and psychometric properties of nine standardized neonatal assessments [1]. Two main trends may be identified among these evaluation tools. Some assessments such as the Brazelton's Neonatal Behavioral Assessment Scale – NBAS [2] and the Assessment of Preterm Infant Behavior – APIB [3] are more behaviour-oriented by emphasizing interactive behaviours between infant and caregiver, neonate's ability to cope with stress and regulatory capacities. Other assessments such as the Test of Infant Motor Performance – TIMP [4] and the Alberta's Infant Motor Scale – AIMS [5] are more motor-oriented by analyzing reflexes, motor patterns, postures and/or volitional movements. Recently, Prechtl and his collaborators have proposed the infant's spontaneous movements as the most meaningful cerebral function to test [6, 7].

Regardless of the type of assessment used during the neonatal period, a normal exam has a good negative predictive value for disability [1]. However, the positive predictive value of such an early measurement of neurological functioning for long term disability is poor, as judged by the published literature. For instance, several studies looking at the relationship between neonatal behaviour, measured with the NBAS, and developmental outcome have found that behavioural organization scores alone account for a significant but small-to-moderate proportion of the variance in outcome [2].

The patterns of change in neonatal behaviour reflect the ability of the neonate to reorganize after experiencing a stressful interaction [2]. Therefore, extreme caution is recommended concerning prediction of a poor outcome based on an early assessment. Multiple and consecutive examinations are much more sensitive to perinatal influences as indices of future organization, than is one examination. The lack of positive predictive value for a poor outcome is not difficult to understand: one reason is "central", as maturation of the hemispheric structures is just beginning; the other is "peripheral", as musculotendinous contractures due to unphysiological postures in the Neonatal Intensive Care Unit (NICU) are often present and may mimic neurological abnormalities.

Neurological assessment at 2 years corrected

The following facts emerge from what is currently known in the VLBW infant concerning the anatomo-physiological correlates and the most usual types of lesions. 1) Anatomo-physiological correlates [8] allow the development of upper (hemispheric) system to be followed from birth to 2 years corrected, by assessing the progressive control exerted on the lower (brainstem) system. Therefore any deficit in this hierarchical organization will be detectable in assessing motor function as well as gross and fine motor development. 2) Brain damage in premature infants is mainly located in hemispheric structures, with cerebral atrophy predominating in periventricular white matter and neuronal loss as well as cicatricial gliosis found in various structures; the brain stem is usually spared. Consequently, dysfunction in upper motor control is expected to be a prominent feature, even if it is associated with signs of dysfunction in areas other than neuromotor. 3) Due to the amazing speed of growth of cerebral hemispheres within the first 2 years, head growth curves and assessment of cranial sutures may provide valuable information [9-11].

A clinical methodology derived from André-Thomas and Saint-Anne-Dargassies has been progressively developed [12, 13] to take into account the facts summarized above. A scoring system is now proposed [14, 15] from birth to 6 years, to obtain a better categorization of neuromotor findings through infancy and childhood. As an example, the NIH Developmental Research Network [16] has been using the Amiel-Tison neurological assessment [15] in conjunction with the Bayley test [17] to evaluate neurodevelopmental and functional outcomes in 1480 VLBW infants at 18 to 22 months' corrected age. In this study, 25% of the children had an abnormal neurological examination including cerebral palsy (CP) diagnosed in 17%. The relationship between Bayley scores and neurological status was evaluated. Most of the children with abnormal neurological findings had a deficient motor function, with a psychomotor developmental index (PDI) more than 2 SD below the norm in 73% of the children; only 14% of the children with a normal neurological examination had a PDI below the norm. Additionally, 69% of children with an abnormal neurological examination had a mental developmental index (MDI) more than 2 SD below the norm compared to 26% of children with a normal neurological examination.

The Amiel-Tison neurological assessment allows a cohort of children to be divided and categorized according to a continuum from severe to mild signs. Categorization is based on the nature and association of neurological and cranial signs, as shown in *table I*. The symptomatic "neuro-cranial triad" including phasic stretch reflex, imbalance of passive tone and presence of squamous ridges, as already studied [10], has recently shown a significant correlation at preschool age [18], not only with coordination but also with reasoning and language. Recent data also suggest a significant association between these signs detected at 2 years of age and IQ, mainly verbal IQ, assessed at 6 years of age in the same cohort of high risk children [19]. These results confirm the frequent association between mild pyramidal findings and lower cognitive functioning in high risk infants.

Table I. Categorization according to the nature and association of neurological and cranial signs.

Categories	Neurological signs
Cerebral Palsy (CP)	Abnormal posture and movements No independent walk by 2 years corrected
Mild spasticity	Uni or bilateral tonic stretch reflex ± other abnormalities Independent walk before 2 years corrected
Neuro-cranial Triad	Uni or bilateral phasic stretch reflex Imbalance of passive axial tone Squamous ridges
Miscellaneous	Minor isolated findings
Normal	No neurological signs

Neuropsychological assessment at 7 to 9 years

If the research goal is to test high cerebral functions and processing, it is necessary to wait until the children reach school age, *i.e.* 7 to 9 years. At this age, the neuropsychological evaluation of children tends to focus on the following domains: attention, perception, memory, language, spatial construction, executive function, motor skills and affect. A fairly extensive battery of tests has to be administered, including measures of affect and personality [20]. The assessment by the psychologist usually includes the Wechsler Intelligence Scale for Children – WISC-IV [21], a widely used test of cognitive function giving a full-scale IQ and separate Verbal and Performance quotients or the Kaufman Assessment Battery for Children (K-ABC) [22]. The K-ABC measures cognitive ability by means of two processing scales: sequential processing or problem-solving by serial or temporal ordering of stimuli, and simultaneous processing which involves a holistic, often spatial integration of stimuli. The K-ABC also includes a separate achievement scale so that ability may be compared with achievement level. Concerning emotional disorders, a wide variety of child behaviour rating scales is available [23].

Proposed strategy for developmental outcome research in VLBW infants

At what age can one expect meaningful differences?

As discussed above, three periods can be described:

Neurological assessment at 40 weeks has a poor positive predictive value for disability. Therefore, in the immediate postnatal period, differences based on extraneurological factors such as weight gain, head growth, length of hospital stay could be the best markers, as already used by Als & Gilkerson [24].

Neurological assessment at 2 years corrected age allows the investigator to split a cohort into 3 groups based on neurological findings. Optimal results are well defined and severe sequelae are diagnosed, including cerebral palsy (CP), severe mental, behavioural, and/or sensory impairments. Identification of a high risk group for later disabilities becomes much more precise, based on neuromotor and cranial findings. In parallel to the neurological assessment, a developmental test such as the new Bayley [17] or the Griffiths [25] should be performed. This approach at 2 years of corrected age is technically feasible, not expensive, and may or may not be sensitive enough to demonstrate the marginal effects of deleterious environmental factors.

At school age, neuropsychological assessment will identify learning disabilities that will correlate with later executive dysfunction at adult age [26]. However, the level of "contamination" by ongoing environmental factors during childhood is so high that factoring out influences of organic *vs.* environmental factors becomes illusive.

Several kinds of difficulties can be expected: 1) tests are time consuming, therefore expensive; 2) the percentage of drop-out is high at this age; 3) children from families that do not speak the native language at home have to be eliminated from the study due to the paramount importance of language in each of the tests used; 4) the socio-familial environment will exert significant influence on school achievement. Therefore, although waiting until school age to measure the potential effects of adverse environmental factors that occurred during the neonatal period seems very wise, it appears at the same time highly unsatisfactory, as other variables including therapeutic interventions and socio-familial environment may prevent the detection of significant and isolated effect.

What choice for a control group?

Ideally, premature newborn infants with and without developmental care should be matched. By experience however, the influence of the study on the nursing staff practices is such that management in the control group (without developmental care) consistently changes during the study period.

To counter this difficulty, the alternative should be to choose the control group in another NICU in which developmental care has not yet been developed. Such a set-up seems very inadequate to demonstrate subtle differences, due to the potential inequality of care in other domains. Whatever the methods selected for assessing the children, the study design remains exceedingly difficult, as stressed in the recent literature [27-29].

Philosophical reasons for developmental care

Developmental care is attractive and makes sense. However several aspects need discussion. For instance, do we expect that adaptive capacities and compensatory mechanisms should be more efficient in children with an intact brain that in those with brain damage? In other words, are the benefits of developmental care to be found in the healthiest premature infants (having preserved their optimal genetic potentialities) or in the brain-damaged children? If developmental care is more effective in the impaired children, it could be impossible to demonstrate that the outcome could even be worse if the effects of an aggressive and disorganized environment are added to the effects of brain damage.

Another question concerns the definition of an intact brain, especially in the Extremely Low Birth Weight (ELBW) group: does the absence of neurological and cranial signs allow us to define an intact brain? Probably not. As seen above, dichotomy between organic and nonorganic etiological factors for late sequelae may be based on the clinical identification of neurological and cranial signs. It may be based as well on imaging and traditional electrophysiological studies. However, we know that owing the extreme immaturity of the brain at birth in the ELBW group, the risk for learning disability is higher than in the general population, even in the absence of neurological findings or abnormal imaging. In fact, subtle disorganization of the brain may be inherent to the lowest gestational age at birth and environmental factors could have an additive effect on this already disorganized brain. The particular level at which a noxious environment may become deleterious remains unknown [24].

Conclusion

As often discussed in scientific circles, methodological limitations are overwhelming: the choice of a control group, blinding, the stability of care in the control group are all sources of difficulties such that many trials have to be stopped before reaching a cohort large enough to provide a significant answer. Considering the worst case scenario, it could happen that no definite answer is possible as to the benefit of developmental care, due to these limitations. However the by-products of such a research program would be very valuable indeed in increasing our understanding of cerebral function in ELBW infants. Studying a cohort from 40 weeks to 7 to 9 years would help us to understand whether the early benefits of developmental care are maintained at school age or vanish under the weight of potential confounders. In any case, one can predict that such studies will have a positive effect on the promotion of developmental care even if we fail to offer an indisputable demonstration of the expected benefits.

In his thoughtful editorial of the January 2001 issue of Developmental Medicine and Child Neurology [30], Martin Bax quotes the 1998 document of the European Academy of Childhood Disability [31]. *"Certain services or facilities should be available as a basic right in a caring society, rather than these having to meet a strict scientific test of effectiveness"*. He then comments on the benefits of physiotherapy in CP children coming up with this insight: *"If we were looking at the effects of therapy, not in term of measures... but more in term of parental satisfaction and ease of management of the child, maybe we would get better results"*. As a caring society, we should provide the greatest care possible to our most vulnerable newcomers.

References

1. Majnemer A, Mazer B. Neurologic evaluation of the newborn infant: definition and psychometric properties. *Dev Med Child Neurol* 1998; 40: 708-15.

2. Brazelton TB, Nugent JK. Neonatal Behavioral Assessment Scale. *Clin Dev Med* 1995: 137.

3. Als H, Lester B, Tronick E, Brazelton TB. Manual for the Assessment of Preterm Infants' Behavior (APIB). In: Fitzgerald H, Lester B, Togman M, eds. *Theory and research in behavioural pediatrics*. New York: Plenum Press, 1982: 65-132.

4. Campbell S, Orten E, Kollobe T, Fisher AG. Development of the test of infant motor performance. *Physical and Medical Rehabilitation Clinics* 1993; 4: 541-50.

5. Piper M, Darrah J. *Motor Assessment of the Developing Infant*. Toronto: WB Saunders Co, 1994.

6. Prechtl HFR, Einspieler C, Cioni G, Bos AF, Ferrari F, Sontheimer D. An early marker for neurological deficits after perinatal brain lesions. *Lancet* 1997; 349: 1361-3.

7. Cioni G, Ferrari F, Einspieler C, Paolicelli PB, Barbani MT, Prechtl HFR. Comparison between observation of spontaneous movements and neurologic examination in preterm infants. *J Pediatr* 1997; 130: 704-11.

8. Sarnat HB. Anatomic and physiologic correlates of neurological development in prematurity. In: Sarnat HB, ed. *Topics in Neonatal Neurology*. Orlando, Florida: Grune and Stratton, 1984: 1-25.

9. Amiel-Tison C, Gosselin J, Infante-Rivard C. Head growth and cranial assessment as part of the neurological examination in infancy. *Dev Med Child Neurol* 2002; 44: 643-8.

10. Amiel-Tison C, Njiokiktjien C, Vaivre-Douret L, Verschoor CA, Chavanne E, Garel M. Relation of early neuromotor and cranial signs with neuropsychological outcome at 4 years. *Brain Dev* 1996; 18: 280-6.

11. Amiel-Tison C, Stewart A. Apparently normal survivors: neuromotor and cognitive function as they grow older. In: Amiel-Tison C, Stewart A, eds. *The newborn infant: One brain for life*. Paris: Editions INSERM, 1994: 227-37.

12. Amiel-Tison C. Neuromotor status. In: Taeusch HW, Yogman MW, eds. *Follow-up management of the high-risk infant*. Boston: Little Brown, 1987: 115-26.

13. Amiel-Tison C, Stewart A. Follow-up studies during the first five years of life: a pervasive assessment of neurological function. *Arch Dis Child* 1989; 64: 496-502.

14. Amiel-Tison C, Gosselin J. *Développement neurologique de la naissance à 6 ans. Manuel et grille d'évaluation*. Montréal: Hôpital Ste Justine, 1998.

15. Amiel-Tison C, Gosselin J. *Neurological Development from Birth to 6 Years: User Manual and Examination Chart*. Baltimore: John Hopkins University, 2001.

16. Vohr BR, Wright LL, Dusick AM, et al. Neurodevelopmental and Functional Outcomes of Extremely Low Birth Weight Infants in the National Institute of Child Health and Human Development Neonatal Research Network. *Pediatrics* 2000; 105: 1216-26.

17. Bayley N. *Bayley Scales in Infant Development II*. San Antonio: Psychological Corporation, 1993.

18. Gosselin J, Amiel-Tison C, Infante-Rivard C, Fouron C, Fouron JC. Minor neurological signs and developmental performance in high risk children at preschool age. *Dev Med Child Neurol* 2002; 44: 323-8.

19. Gosselin J, Amiel-Tison C. Évaluation de la fonction neuromotrice de la naissance à 6 ans. Catégorisation à 2 ans d'âge corrigé. Corrélation avec le QI à 6 ans. *Progrès en néonatalogie*. Paris: Société Française de Néonatologie, 2004: 15-28.

20. Mattis S. Neuropsychological assessment of school-aged children. In: Rapin I, Segalowitz SJ, eds. *Handbook of neuropsychology, vol. 6*. Amsterdam: Elsevier, 1992: 395-415.

21. Wechsler D. *Wechsler Intelligence Scales for Children*. New York: Psychological Corporation, 1974.

22. Kaufman AS. *Kaufman Assessment Battery for Children*. Circle Pines: American Guidance, 1983.

23. Barkley RA. Child behavior rating scales and checklists. In: Rutter M, Tuma AH, Lann IS, eds. *Assessment and Diagnosis in Child Psychopathology*. New York: Guilford Press, 1987: 115-55.

24. Als H, Gilkerson L. The role of relationship-based developmentally supportive newborn intensive care in strengthening outcome of preterm infants. *Semin Perinatol* 1997; 21: 178-89.

25. Griffiths R. *The abilities of young children*. Buck. The Test Agency Ltd, 1954.

26. Bridge Denckla M. The child with developmental disabilities grown-up: adult residua of childhood disorders. In: Brumback RA, guest ed. *Neurologic Clinics Behavioral Neurology* 1993; 11: 105-25.

27. Aylward G, Pfeiffer S. Follow-up and outcome of low-birth-weight infants: conceptual issues and a methodology review. *Aust Pediatr J* 1989; 25: 3-5.

28. Bellinger D, Leviton A, Stiles K. Developmental disorders of cerebral function: epidemiological principles and pitfalls. In: Rapin I, Segalowitz SJ, eds. *Handbook of neuropsychology*. Amsterdam: Elsevier, 1992: 211-22.

29. Mc Cormick MC. The outcomes of very low birth weight infants: are we asking the right questions. *Pediatrics* 1997; 99: 869-76.

30. Bax M. Does "therapy" have a future? *Dev Med Child Neurol* 2001; 43: 3-3.

31. Mc Conachie H, Smyth D, Bax M. Services for children with disabilities in European countries. *Dev Med Child Neurol* 1997; 39 (suppl. 76): 5.

Electroencephalography and developmental care

Lena Hellström-Westas, Ingmar Rosén

The electroencephalogram (EEG) in the mature brain is a spatiotemporal average of synchronous post-synaptic potentials in cortical pyramidal cells oriented in parallel. Synchronous neuronal activity arises by several mechanisms. Individual thalamocortical relay cells, cells in the thalamic reticular nucleus and cortical pyramidal cells each have endogenous recurrent action potential firing properties [1]. The activity within groups of thalamocortical neurons is synchronised by recurrent connections between thalamocortical relay cells and the surrounding reticular thalamic nucleus, and between the thalamus and cortex. During arousal, cholinergic (and noradrenergic) afferents from the brainstem exert an excitatory depolarizing effect on thalamocortical and cortical cells and inhibit the reticular thalamus. The net result of arousal is a reduction of synchronous activity and an increase of asynchronous high-frequency activity.

The main mechanisms for the generation of EEG are probably relevant for the full-term newborn, but our knowledge about EEG mechanisms in the immature brain of the extremely preterm infant are more limited. However, since EEG has been recorded also in many extremely preterm infants there is good knowledge about normal maturational changes and characteristics of abnormal changes [2, 3]. The EEG of a stable extremely preterm infant is discontinuous, *i.e.* periods of relative quiescence (low amplitude) are mixed with periods with those of higher amplitude. During maturation the EEG background becomes increasingly continuous, and interhemispheric synchronisation increases [4-6]. The EEG contains specific features that are typical and normal for a certain gestational age but can be abnormal at other maturational levels, *e.g.* "delta brushes", that is, slow (delta) activity with superimposed fast (beta) activity occurring first at around 30 weeks gestation and with a distribution that changes with increasing maturation [7]. Sleep wake cycling can usually be identified in the EEG at 29-30 weeks gestation, although cyclical changes suggestive of sleep wake cycling are discernible in the amplitude integrated EEG (aEEG) of well infants with postmenstrual ages as low as 25-26 weeks [8, 9].

The amplitude-integrated EEG (aEEG) is a method for continuous monitoring of electrocortical brain activity. The method was constructed with the aims of being simple to use and interpret in the NICU, and to create minimal disturbances for the patients. The aEEG records a single (or two) channel EEG, with an asymmetric band-pass filter that includes the main EEG-frequencies. The recorded EEG undergoes rectification and smoothing before it is displayed as a semilogarithmic time-compressed signal, either written onto paper (*e.g.* Cerebral Function Monitor, CFM

Multitrace™), or displayed on a computer screen (*e.g.* Nicolet One™, Olympic CFM 6000™, Brainz monitor™, or the Cerebral Function Analyzing Monitor, CFAM™) [10]. The aEEG has been used in preterm infants for evaluation of cerebral activity in relation to intracranial haemorrhages, and for evaluating effects from certain medications such as surfactant and morphine [11, 12].

The background EEG in the full-term infant is a strong predictor of neurological outcome when recorded early after an insult, *e.g.* perinatal asphyxia [13]. The early EEG of the extremely preterm infant is also clearly related to the degree of acute intracerebral pathology [14-16]. However, in extremely preterm infants the correlation between early EEG and outcome is not as clear as in the full-term infants since outcome is affected by several factors that are primarily non-neurological, *e.g.* nutrition, late-onset sepsis and bronchopulmonary dysplasia (BPD) [17].

Acute changes in the EEG and aEEG

Major acute abnormalities in the EEGs of preterm infants include increased discontinuity and presence of epileptic seizure activity. There are other, and more subtle, chronic changes that may appear in the EEG during abnormal conditions. One such example is presence of positive rolandic sharp waves (PRSW) that are markers of cerebral white matter injury. An increased number of PRSW is associated with an increased risk for developing cerebral palsy [18]. This overview will focus on acute changes in the EEG, and aEEG, which are associated with specific clinical situations occurring in preterm infants.

• Development of intraventricular (germinal matrix) haemorrhages (IVH) and periventricular leukomalacia (PVL) is associated with initial depression of the EEG background and presence of epileptic seizure activity [8, 14, 19-21]. There is a clear correlation between the number of damaged brain structures in preterm infants and degree of EEG abnormality [22]. The electrocortical background usually recovers within the first week of life in infants with IVH; the rate of this recovery is predictive of gross neurological outcome in preterm infants with large IVH's, as recorded with aEEG [23]. Epileptic seizures are common in infants developing IVH and PVL [8, 14, 21]. The seizures are often subclinical, but the presence of seizure activity does not seem to be related to outcome [23]. A measure of EEG, the spectral edge frequency (SEF) seems to be predictive of white matter injury in very low birthweight preterm infants [24].

• Several medications can depress EEG activity in preterm infants. These medications include phenobarbitone, diazepam, morphine, sufentanil and surfactant [11, 12, 22, 25, 26]. Consequently, when evaluating the EEG of preterm infants, effects from medications must be taken into account. Administration of surfactant and diazepam to preterm infants often results in a marked, but relatively short, depression of the EEG or aEEG amplitude [11, 23]. The response to phenobarbital and morphine is usually more sustained but milder [12]. Possible direct effects on the preterm infant's EEG from some of the commonly used medications such as indomethacin and theophyllamine have not, to our knowledge, been evaluated.

- Blood exchange transfusions may cause transient mild depression in the aEEG which is related to blood pressure changes [27]. One study in preterm infants indicated that metabolic and respiratory acidosis was associated with a reversible increase in EEG discontinuity [28]. Acid-base changes and some care procedures should consequently be regarded when interpreting EEG in preterm infants.

- Effects from pain on the neonatal EEG have only been described in a few studies, mainly including studies on newborn animals. The response on EEG from oral sucrose versus oral water was evaluated in full-term newborn infants who were exposed to a "heelstroke", a noxious but non-invasive procedure included in the Neonatal Behavioral Assessment Scale (NBAS) [29]. Infants who received water, but not infants who received sucrose, showed increased right frontal EEG activation (3 to 6 Hz frequency), a pattern associated with negative affect [30]. Preterm infants also exhibit clear responses to pain, and it is possible that pain responses could be measured with EEG. However, to our knowledge there are no studies evaluating the acute EEG in relation to pain or stress in preterm infants.

- The quality of sleep in preterm infants is affected by several factors, *e.g.* external time cues such as feeding schedules, thermal environment, and positioning of the infant. Sleep in preterm infants can be quantified in various ways, *e.g.* total sleep time, longest sleep time, duration and amount of quiet and active sleep, as measured by EEG or by clinical observation. Sleep wake cycling is often disturbed in newborn infants during intensive care often due to sedative medications, but also due to circumstances with affected brain function. The aEEG has been used for studying acute effects on sleep from incubator covers and developmental care in preterm infants [31, 32]. Minor changes related to the interventions were detected during quiet sleep, which is the only sleep parameter that is possible to evaluate with aEEG. Hence, this method does not allow evaluation of other sleep parameters where more evident changes might have occurred.

The aEEG can be used for on-line monitoring of electrocortical brain activity for days (and weeks when necessary). *Figures 1 to 4* show examples of aEEG traces from extremely preterm infants in various clinical situations (normal, surfactant, morphine, replated care procedures).

Chronic changes in the EEG

Both acute and chronic changes in the EEG background correlated with later neurological outcome. Acute changes in the EEG background, *e.g.* amplitude depression and seizures are usually relatively easy to diagnose while chronic changes usually are more subtle. Chronic changes include poor organization of the electricocortical background activity and poor organization of sleep wake states, as well as presence of abnormal wave forms, *e.g.* positive rolandic sharp waves (PRSW). Depending on the nature of the chronic EEG changes, they can be related to risk for abnormal cognitive development and development of abnormal neurological conditions, *e.g.* cerebral palsy. As mentioned above, PRSW are relatively late appearing signs related to white matter injury in prematurely born infants. Marret *et al.* showed that there was a correlation between presence of more than two PRSW per second in the EEG's of preterm infants and

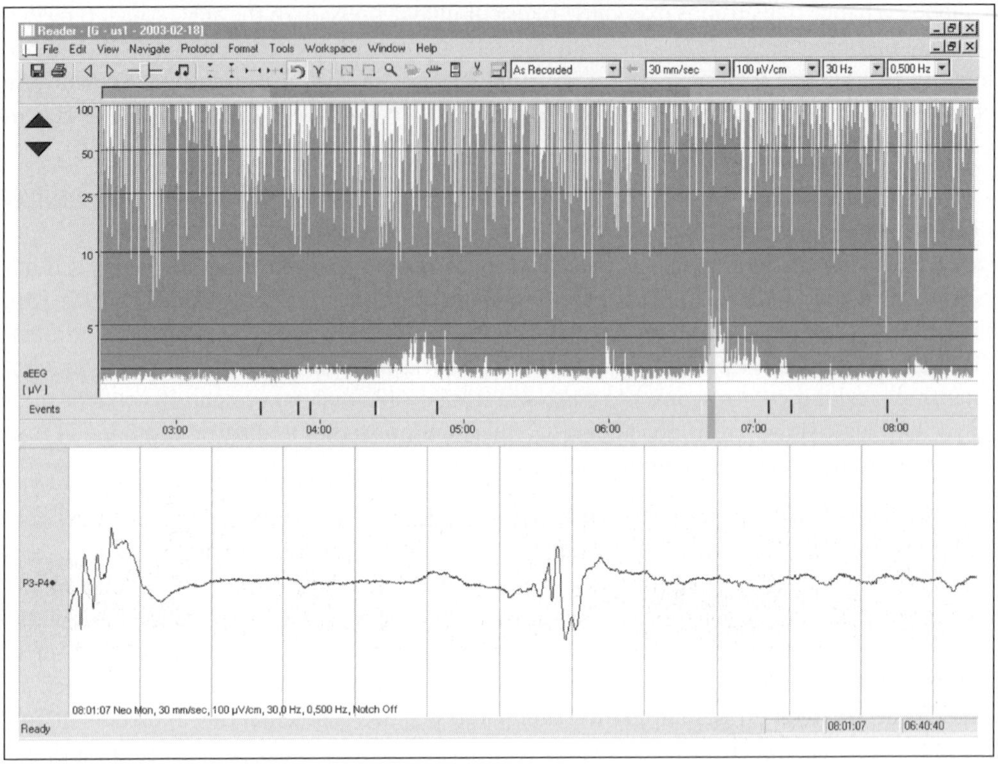

Figure 1. Normal discontinuous aEEG recording with some variability from a two day old infant of 25 weeks gestation. The infant was mechanically ventilated and sedated with morphine. Cranial ultrasound was normal. The duration of the aEEG recording (upper tracing) is six hours. The lower tracing shows 12 seconds of simultaneously recorded EEG activity with a tracé discontinue pattern.

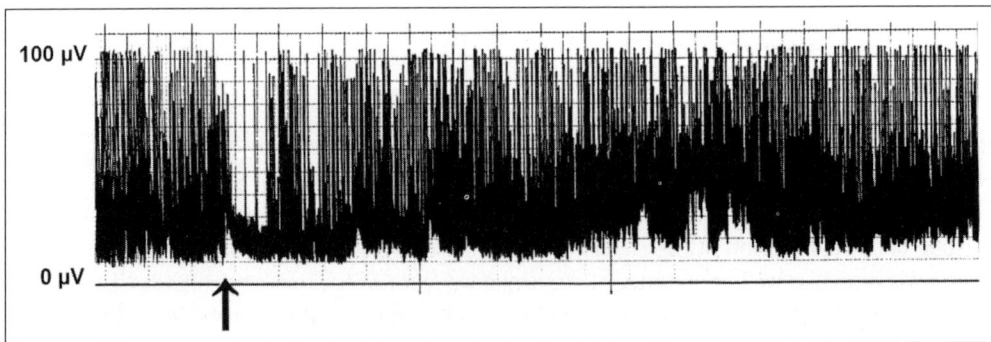

Figure 2. Amplitude integrated EEG recording showing transient depression of cerebroelectrical activity after surfactant administration (arrow) in an extremely preterm infant. The cerebral activity recovers after 10 minutes and there are no other abnormalities in the tracing. The total duration of the recording is 3 hours 20 minutes. Hellström-Westas et al., with permission from Parthenon Publishing.

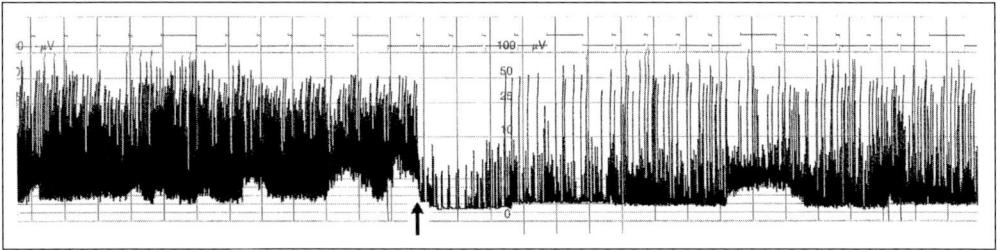

Figure 3. Decrease in cerebral activity after administration of morphine (arrow) in a stable, 30-week gestation, infant on mechanical ventilation after a blood exchange transfusion due to Rhesus immunization. The reaction to morphine is unusually marked in this infant. The reason for this is unknown, but could be a signal that the infant was more fragile than was clinically recognised. The duration of this recording is almost 5 hours with 10 minutes between the vertical lines. Hellström-Westas et al., with permission from Parthenon Publishing.

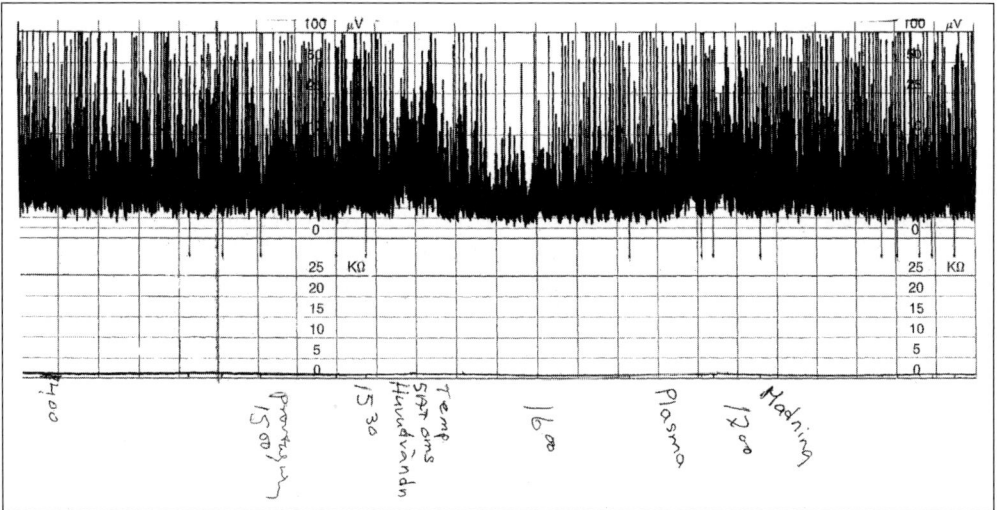

Figure 4. Subtle decrease in cerebral activity during 30 minutes after repeated care procedures (notes below the tracing), as shown by the decrease in burst rate in the middle of this 4-hour aEEG tracing from a 25 week gestation infant. Hellström-Westas et al., with permission from Parthenon Publishing.

development of cerebral palsy [18]. The aEEG, which is excellent for long-term monitoring of changes in electrocortical background activity including sleep-wake cycling, does not show subtle EEG features, *e.g.* presence of sharp waves or PRSW.

• Delayed maturation is present when presence of developmental milestones in the EEG is delayed with more than 2-3 weeks. This is a nonspecific sign that is associated with increased risk for adverse outcome. Delayed maturation of the EEG is common in infants with BPD. The distribution of EEG frequencies over the hemispheres can be visually displayed by *e.g.* brain mapping. In a randomized controlled study on effects from NIDCAP treatment, Buehler *et al.* found that the infants who were assigned NIDCAP treatment had signs of increased maturation on brain mapping EEG at full-term than control infants [33].

- Synchronisation of cerebroelectrical activity increases during maturation, although lack of, or delayed, synchronisation are nonspecific abnormal signs. Coherence is a measure of synchronisation of activity between different brain regions. Our knowledge about normal coherence in the neonatal period is limited, since the method requires advanced programs for EEG analysis. However, preliminary data suggests that preterm infants who received developmental care according to NIDCAP at full-term had higher fronto-occipital EEG coherence as compared to control infants [34].

- The quality and quantity of sleep can be measured with EEG after around 30 weeks gestation. Some qualities of sleep are related to brain maturation and differ between full-term and prematurely born infants when recorded with EEG at the same maturational level [35]. Some sleep-parameters can also be associated with cognitive outcome [36]. Sleep is discussed more in another chapter.

Conclusion

The EEG is a sensitive tool for detecting acute and chronic cerebral dysfunction, and for gross prediction of outcome in preterm infants. Several care procedures as well as medications that are used during the intensive care period may affect the acute EEG/aEEG and make the interpretation more difficult. There is only limited information regarding EEG responses to stress and pain in newborn infants, although recent data suggests that EEG could be an additional tool for investigating pain responses. New advanced EEG methods for evaluating sleep quality and coherence are likely to become valuable for research on developmental care and add to our knowledge on mechanisms for cognitive dysfunction in prematurely born infants.

References

1. Steriade M, Gloor P, Llinás RR, Lopes da Silva FH, Mesulam MM. Report of IFCN committe on basic mechanisms. Basic mechanisms of cerebral rhythmic activities. *Electroencephalogr Clin Neurophysiol* 1990; 76: 481-508.

2. Monod N, Pajot N, Guidasci S. The neonatal EEG: Statistical studies and prognostic value in full-term and preterm babies. *Electroencephalogr Clin Neurophysiol* 1972; 32: 529-44.

3. Lombroso CT. Neonatal polygraphy in full-term and premature infants: a review of normal and abnormal findings. *J Clin Neurophysiol* 1985; 2: 105-55.

4. Lamblin MD, Andre M, Challamel MJ, et al. Electroencephalography of the premature and term newborn. Maturational aspects and glossary. *Neurophysiol Clin* 1999; 29: 123-219.

5. Selton D, Andre M, Hascoet JM. Normal EEG in very premature infants: reference criteria. *Clin Neurophysiol* 2000; 111: 2116-24.

6. Connell JA, Oozeer R, Dubowitz V. Continuous 4-channel EEG monitoring: A guide to interpretation, with normal values, in preterm infants. *Neuropediatrics* 1987; 18: 138-45.

7. Hayakawa M, Okumura A, Hayakawa F, et al. Background electroencephalographic (EEG) activities of very preterm infants born at less than 27 weeks gestation: a study on the degree of continuity. *Arch Dis Child Fetal Neonatal Ed* 2001; 84: F163-F167.

8. Hellström-Westas L, Rosén I, Svenningsen NW. Cerebral function monitoring in extremely small low birth-weight (ESLBW) infants during the first week of life. *Neuropediatrics* 1991; 22: 27-32.

9. Kuhle S, Klebermass K, Olischar M, *et al*. Sleep-wake cycling in preterm infants below 30 weeks of gestational age. Preliminary results of a prospective amplitude-integrated EEG study. *Wien Klin Wochenschr* 2001; 113: 219-23.

10. Prior P, Maynard DE. *Monitoring cerebral function. Long-term recordings of cerebral electrical activity and evoked potentials*. Amsterdam: Elsevier, 1986: 1-441.

11. Hellström-Westas L, Bell AH, Skov L, Greisen G, Svenningsen NW. Cerebroelectrical depression following surfactant treatment in preterm neonates. *Pediatrics* 1992; 89: 643-47.

12. Bell AH, Greisen G, Pryds O. Comparison of the effects of phenobarbitone and morphine administration on EEG activity in preterm babies. *Acta Paediatr* 1993; 82: 35-9.

13. Holmes G, Rowe J, Hafford J, Schmidt R, Testa M, Zimmerman A. Prognostic value of the electroencephalogram in neonatal asphyxia. *Electroencephalogr Clin Neurophysiol* 1982; 53: 60-72.

14. Connell J, Oozeer R, Regev R, de Vries LS, Dubowitz LMS, Dubowitz V. Continuous four-channel EEG monitoring in the evaluation of echodense ultrasound lesions and cystic leukomalacia. *Arch Dis Child* 1987; 62: 1019-24.

15. Biagioni E, Bartalena L, Biver P, Pieri R, Cioni G. Electroencephalographic dysmaturity in preterm infants: a prognostic tool in the early postnatal period. *Neuropediatrics* 1996; 27: 311-6.

16. Watanabe K, Hayakawa F, Okumura A. Neonatal EEG: a powerful tool in the assessment of brain damage in preterm infants. *Brain Dev* 1999; 21: 361-72.

17. Tharp BR, Scher MS, Clancy RR. Serial EEGs in normal and abnormal infants with birthweights less than 1200 grams – a prospective study with long term follow-up. *Neuropediatrics* 1989; 20: 64-72.

18. Marret S, Parain D, Ménard J-F, *et al*. Prognostic value of neonatal electroencephalography in premature newborns less than 33 weeks gestational age. *Electroencephalogr Clin Neurophsysiol* 1997; 102: 178-85.

19. Watanabe K, Hakamada S, Kuroyanagi M, Yamazaki T, Takeuchi T. Electroencephalographical study of intraventricular hemorrhage in the preterm infant. *Neuropediatrics* 1983; 14: 225-30.

20. Clancy RR, Tharp BR, Enzman D. EEG in premature infants with intraventricular hemorrhage. *Neurology* 1984; 34: 583-90.

21. Greisen G, Hellström-Westas L, Lou H, Rosén I, Svenningsen NW. EEG depression and germinal layer haemorrhage in the newborn. *Acta Paediatr Scand* 1987; 76: 519-25.

22. Aso K, Abdad-Barmada M, Scher MS. EEG and the neuropathology in premature neonates with intraventricular hemorrhage. *J Clin Neurophysiol* 1993; 10: 304-13.

23. Hellström-Westas L, Klette H, Thorngren-Jerneck K, Rosén I. Early prediction of outcome with aEEG in preterm infants with large intraventricular hemorrhages. *Neuropediatrics* 2001; 32: 319-24.

24. Inder TE, Buckland L, Williams CE, *et al*. Lowered electroencephalographic spectral edge frequency predicts the presence of cerebral white matter injury in premature infants. *Pediatrics* 2003; 111: 27-33.

25. Young GB, da Silva OP. Effects of morphine on the electroencephalograms of neonates: a prospective, observational study. *Clin Neurophysiol* 2000; 111: 1955-60.

26. Nguyen The Tich S, Vecchierini MF, Debillon T, Pereon Y. Effects of sufentanil on electroencephalogram in very and extremely preterm neonates. *Pediatrics* 2003; 111: 123-8.

27. Benders MJ, Meinesz JH, van Bel F, van de Bor M. Changes in electrocortical brain activity during exchange transfusions in newborn infants. *Biol Neonate* 2000; 78: 17-21.

28. Eaton DG, Wertheim D, Oozeer R, Dubowitz LM, Dubowitz V. Reversible changes in cerebral activity associated with acidosis in preterm neonates. *Acta Paediatr* 1994; 83: 486-92.

29. Brazelton TB. The Brazelton Neonatal Behavior Assessment Scale: introduction. *Monogr Soc Res Child Dev* 1978; 43: 1-13.

30. Fernandez M, Blass EM, Hernandez-Reif M, Field T, Diego M, Sanders C. Sucrose attenuates a negative electroencephalographic response to an aversive stimulus for newborns. *J Dev Behav Pediatr* 2003; 24: 261-6.

31. Hellström-Westas L, Inghammar M, Isaksson K, Rosén I, Stjernqvist K. Short-term effects of incubator covers on quiet sleep in stable premature infants. *Acta Paediatr* 2001; 90: 1004-8.

32. Westrup B, Hellström-Westas L, Stjernqvist K, Lagercrantz H. No indications of increased quiet sleep in infants receiving care based on the newborn individualized developmental care and assessment program (NIDCAP). *Acta Paediatr* 2002; 91: 318-22.

33. Buehler DM, Als H, Duffy FH, McAnulty GB, Liederman J. Effectiveness of individualized developmental care for low-risk preterm infants: behavioral and electrophysiologic evidence. *Pediatrics* 1995; 96: 923-32.

34. Als A, Duffy FH, McAnulty G, *et al*. Early Experience Alters Brain Function and Structure. *Pediatrics* 2004 113: 846-57.

35. Scher MS, Sun M, Steppe DA, Banks DL, Guthrie RD, Sclabassi RJ. Comparisons of EEG sleep state-specific spectral values between healthy full-term and preterm infants at comparable postconceptional ages. *Sleep* 1994; 17: 47-51.

36. Scher MS, Steppe DA, Banks DL. Prediction of lower developmental performances of healthy neonates by neonatal EEG-sleep measures. *Pediatr Neurol* 1996; 14: 137-44.

Cerebral Near Infrared Spectroscopy. A useful tool for developmental care research?

Gorm Greisen

Transillumination of the head of small animals is possible using near infrared spectroscopy (NIRS). The first clinical research use of NIRS in 1985 was in human newborns [1]. Quantitative spectroscopy was subsequently performed in 1986 [2]. Over the following years many papers on NIRS in newborns have been published. The purpose of the present paper is to provide a short overview and discuss the potential use of NIRS for improving the scientific basis of developmental care.

NIRS methodology

Geometry

The newborn infant's head is ideally suited for NIRS. The overlying tissues are relatively thin which ensures that the signal is dominated by brain tissue, white as well as grey matter. NIRS recordings can be performed with the light applied to one side of the head and received on the other side (transmission mode) in the low-birth-weight infants with biparietal diameters from 6 to 8 cms. In this situation a large part of the brain is "seen" during the measurement, and the results may be interpreted as "global". Larger babies can only be investigated with the emitting and receiving fibres in an angular arrangement (reflection mode), possibly with both on the same side of the head. In this situation a smaller volume of tissue between the optodes is seen, which may be chosen on purpose. It also may be chosen for smaller babies to obtain "regional" results. With a shorter interoptode distance, a more narrow and more shallow tissue volume is seen with a relatively larger fraction of extracerebral tissues. Therefore, distances of less than 4 cms are not recommended.

Algorithms

Several different types of NIRS instruments have been used. The number of wavelengths used has varied from 2 to 6. The specific wavelengths used, and therefore the mathematical algorithms used to separate the signals of oxyhaemoglobin (O2Hb), deoxyhaemoglobin (HHb), and the cytochrome aa3 oxidase difference signal (Cyt.ox), have differed [3]. It is therefore not trivial to ensure that differences in results are not simply due to differences in NIRS methodology, particularly in the earlier papers.

Pathlength

The pathlength of light traversing the tissue must be known to calculate concentrations, that is, to measure quantitatively. The pathlength in tissue exceeds the geometrical distance between the optodes by a factor 3-6 (this factor is the differential path length factor, DPF). Estimation of pathlength is one of the basic problems in NIRS.

Measurements in infants

Trend monitoring of haemoglobin signals

Near infrared spectroscopy is a perfect candidate for use as a clinical monitor of the tiny, sick preterm neonate. It is non-invasive, gives real-time information, does not interfere with intensive care, does not affect the underlying skin and does not remove the infants from the nursery.

In principle NIRS allows on-line trending of changes in O2Hb and HHb, and hence of tHb (the sum of [O2Hb] and [HHb]), which is proportional to changes in cerebral blood volume. This measurement in turn can be used as a surrogate measure of cerebral blood flow. However, the appropriateness of this measure has only been established for reactions to changes in arterial carbondioxide tension [4]. Furthermore, constant optode distance is crucial; if head circumference change even by a fraction of a millimeter as a result of change in brain blood or brain water content, the trends are significantly biased. Minor changes in optode-skin contact induces large transients in the signal and/or baseline shifts.

The difference between [O2Hb] and [HHb] (called Hbdiff, and when divided by a factor of 2 is called oxygen index, OI) is an indicator of the mean oxygen saturation of the haemoglobin in all types of blood vessels in the tissue. This quantity has been shown to change appropriately in many experimental and clinical studies, but has important limitations. Firstly, in terms of interpretation, it is not known how much of the signal comes from blood in arteries, capillaries, and veins, respectively. Recent observations in piglets suggest that the arterial-to-venous ratio is about 1:2 [5]. Secondly, the signal is confounded when there are concomitant changes in tHb, dependent on which of the arterial, capillary, or venous compartments are changed. Finally, the lack of a fixed zero-point makes it impossible to specify a threshold for intervention or even an alarm level for clinical use.

Quantitation of haemoglobin oxygenation

The detection of transmitted light at two or more different distances from the light emitting optodes allows monitoring of the ratio of absolute [O2Hb] to [tHb], *i.e.* the haemoglobin saturation, called "tissue oxygenation index" (TOI). This measure is the weighted average of arterial, capillary and venous blood oxygenation, and hence cannot easily be validated. The measurement depends on the tissue being optically homogeneous, which is unlikely to be the case. Nevertheless, measurements near cerebrovenous values and appropriate changes have been found with changing arterial oxygen saturation, and with arterial pCO2. The signal-to-noise ratio is not as good as that of OI, and hence for quantifying response to brief stimuli TOI is less useful.

Quantitation of cerebral blood volume (CBV)

The effect of a small induced change in arterial oxygen saturation SaO2 on [HbO2] may be used to quantify CBV [6] based on the indicator dilution principle. It is assumed that a small change in arterial oxygen saturation within the normal range will not significantly influence cerebral blood volume, flow or oxygen consumption.

$$[tHb] = 100 \times (\Delta[HbO2] - \Delta[Hb]) / (2 \times \Delta SaO2) \text{ (in μmol/L)}$$

if SaO2 is expressed in %. The total cerebral haemoglobin is directly proportional to the cerebral blood volume:

$$CBV = k \times [tHb] \text{ (in mL/100 g)}$$

where $k = 100 / (Hb \times R \times 1.05)$, Hb is the blood haemoglobin content in mmol/l (tetrahaeme), R is the cerebral-to-large vessel haematocrit ratio, usually taken as 0.69 and the factor 1.05 g/mL is the brain density.

Values for CBV obtained by NIRS in infants are lower than those reported in adults. One explanation could be the lower cerebral blood flow in newborn infants compared to adults. Changes in CBV, induced by bilateral jugular venous occlusion for 5 s, as estimated by NIRS using tHb correlated well with strain gauge plethysmography [7]. This result remains one of the few external quantitative validations of NIRS in the neonatal brain.

Quantitation of cerebral blood flow (CBF)

Measurement of blood flow by NIRS is based on Fick's principle [8] and uses a rapid change in arterial oxyhaemoglobin as an intravascular tracer. By using the change in OI observed after a small sudden change in arterial concentration of oxygen CBF can be calculated as followed:

$$CBF = \Delta OI / (k \times \int SaO2 \times dt), \text{ (in mL/100 g/min)}$$

where OI is measured in units of mol/L, and k = Hb × 1.05 × 100, Hb is blood haemoglobin in mmol/L (tetrahaeme), SaO2 is in %, and t is time in minutes.

The method of measuring CBF rests on several assumptions. Firstly, during measurement CBF, CBV and oxygen extraction must be constant. Secondly, the period of measurement must be less than the cerebral transit time (approx. 10 s). Finally, this method of CBF measurement has practical limitations: In infants with severe lung disease, the SaO2 may be fixed at a low level despite administration of oxygen whereas in infants with normal lungs SaO2 is near 100%, even in room air. This can be overcome by using air-nitrogen mixtures and then switching to room air.

Measurements of blood flow with NIRS have been compared to 133Xe clearance in sick newborn infants. These comparisons constitute important direct external validation of NIRS in the brain of human neonates. The agreement between the two methods is acceptable [9, 10].

Quantitation of cerebro-venous oxygen saturation

Cerebral venous haemoglobin saturation reflects the balance between O2 delivery and O2 consumption. A normal cerebral venous oxygen saturation demonstrates an intact coupling between CBF and the metabolic needs. During restricted blood flow, enhanced oxygen extraction is expected to occur and to result in a drop of cerebro-venous saturation.

Cerebral venous oxygen content may be estimated by near infrared spectrophotometry [2]. When venous outflow from the brain is impeded by tilting head down or by jugular venous occlusion [tHb] increases. Assuming that this is due exclusively to pooling of blood in venoles and veins, cerebral SvO2 can be measured using the formula:

$$cSvO2 = 100 \times \Delta[HbO2] / (\Delta[HbO2] + \Delta[Hb]) \text{ (in \%)}$$

The non-invasive method of measuring cSvO2 with partial jugular venous occlusion was validated with an invasive measurement of SvO2 from co-oximetry of jugular bulb blood obtained during cardiac catherisation and gave similar values [11].

Cytochrome aa3 oxidase

Reduction of cytochrome may be a specific indicator of inadequate cellular O2 availability. We do not know at present, however, with any precision, the relation between tissue pO2, cytochrome oxidation state, and neuronal function. Furthermore, the measurement of cytochrome oxidase with optical techniques is by no means as easy as that of haemoglobin. Firstly, the cytochrome signal is at most one tenth of the haemoglobin signal in amplitude [12]. Secondly, the *in vivo* spectrum is determined by animal experimentation which at the first attempts was complicated by residual haemoglobin signals and by agonal swelling of cells and subcellular elements which influences scattering. Thirdly, there is no reference method.

Optical imaging / multi-regional monitoring

By the use of two or more optodes regional information may be compared, to distinguish between general, systemic responses to stimuli, *e.g.* due to fluctuation in arterial blood pressure or ventilation, from regional responses, *e.g.* due to focal neuronal activation. Neuronal activation is associated with a rapid vasodilatation, to meet the increased metabolic needs and oxygen uptake with increased oxygen supply. In fact, the vasodilation precedes and overshoots the needs, and as a result, [O2Hb] increases as detectable by NIRS and [HHb] decreases as detectable by the BOLD-effect using functional magnetic resonance imaging. Whereas neuronal activation in healthy adults is always associated with focal hyperoxygenation, the vascular reaction in newborns appear less robust, so the oxygenation reaction may be absent or even inverse [13-16].

NIRS and developmental care

Multi-regional monitoring is particularly relevant for developmental care. Visual, olfactory, and proprio-sensory stimuli has been demonstrated to elicite focal hyperoxygenation [13, 17-19]. The signal-to-noise ratio is unfavorable, and averaging of many responses may be necessary. This is time-consuming and has not routinely been done. In principle, sensory thresholds may be determined using NIRS as an objective method. Objective measures of pain and stress is of greater direct relevance to developmental care. It has yet to be shown that NIRS is of use for this specific purpose. One study failed to demonstrate an effect of sucrose before heal lancing on global CBV [20]. A potential problem is that it is expected that systemic circulatory effects of pain and stress may confound the cerebral responses. If a well-defined pattern of (predominant) focal activation could be established, NIRS could become a sensitive tool.

Conclusion and the future

NIRS has matured as a method to obtain quantitative measures of cerebral blood volume, flow and oxygenation and has yielded credible and sometimes important information. The simplest and potentially most practically useful parameter, the oxygenation index, may be confounded by a number of factors. Hyperoxygenation of the primary sensory cortex has been demonstrated in newborn infants using various sensory stimuli, but this response does not appear as robust as in healthy adults. Careful studies, using repeated measurements in individual babies are required to firmly establish the sensitivity of NIRS to detect evoked brain responses.

References

1. Brazy JE, Lewis DV, Mitnisk MH, Jöbsis FF. Non-invasive monitoring of cerebral oxygenation in preterm infants: preliminary observation. *Pediatrics* 1985; 75: 217-25.

2. Wyatt JS, Cope M, Delpy DT, Wray S, Reynolds EOR. Quantification of cerebral oxygenation and haemodynamics in sick newborn infants by near infrared spectrophotometry. *Lancet* 1986; 2: 1063-6.

3. Matcher SJ, Elwell CE, Cooper CE, Cope M, Delpy DT. Performance of several published tissue near infrared spectroscopy algorithms. *Anal Biochem* 1995; 227: 54-68.

4. Pryds O, Greisen G, Skov L, Friis-Hansen B. Carbon dioxide-related changes in cerebral blood volume and cerebral blood flow in mechanically ventilated preterm neonates: comparison of near infrared spectrophotometry and 133Xenon clearance. *Pediatr Res* 1990; 27: 445-9.

5. Brun NC, Moen A, Borch K, Saugstad OD, Greisen G. Near-infrared monitoring of cerebral tissue oxygen saturation and blood volume in newborn piglets. *Am J Physiol* 1997; 273: H682-6.

6. Wyatt JS, Cope M, Delpy DT, van der Zee P, Arridge S, Edwards AD, Reynolds EOR. Quantitation of cerebral blood volume in newborn infants by near infrared spectroscopy. *J Appl Physiol* 1990; 68: 1086-91.

7. Wickramasinghe YABD, Livera LN, Spencer SA, Rolfe P, Thorniley MS. Plethysmographic validation of near infrared spectroscopic monitoring of cerebral blood volume. *Arch Dis Child* 1992; 67: 407-11.

8. Edwards AD, Wyatt JS, Richardson CE, Delpy DT, Cope M, Reynolds EOR. Cotside measurement of cerebral blood flow in ill newborn infants by near-infrared spectroscopy. *Lancet* 1988; 2: 770-1.

9. Skov L, Pryds O, Greisen G. Estimation cerebral blood flow in newborn infants: Comparison of near infrared spectroscopy and 133Xe clearance. *Pediatr Res* 1991; 30, 570-3.

10. Bucher HU, Edwards AD, Lipp AE, Duc G. Comparison between near infrared spectroscopy and 133Xenon clearance for estimation of cerebral blood flow in critically ill preterm infants. *Pediat Res* 1993; 33: 56-60.

11. Yoxall CW, Weindling AM, Dawani NH, Peart I. Measurement of cerebral venous oxyhaemoglobin saturation in children by near infrared spectroscopy and partial jugular venous occlusion. *Pediatr Res* 1995; 38: 319-23.

12. Cope M, van der Zee P, Essenpreis M, Arridge SR, Delpy DT. Data analysis methods for near infrared spectroscopy of tissue: Problems in determining the relative cytochrome aa3 concentration. *Proc SPIE* 1991; 1431: 251-62.

13. Meek JH, Firbank M, Elwell CE, Atkinson J, Braddick O, Wyatt JS. Regional hemodynamic responses to visual stimulation in awake infants. *Pediatr Res* 1998; 43: 840-3.

14. Born P, Leth H, Miranda MJ, Rostrup E, Stensgaard A, Peitersen B, Larsson HB, Lou HC. Visual activation in infants and young children studied by functional magnetic resonance imaging. *Pediatr Res* 1998; 44: 578-83.

15. Taga G, Asakawa K, Maki A, Konishi Y, Koizumi H. Brain imaging in awake infants by near-infrared optical topography. *PNAS* 2003; 100: 10722-7.

16. Konishi Y, Taga G, Yamada H, Hirasawa K. Functional brain imaging using fMRI and optical topography in infancy. *Sleep Med* 2002; 3: S41-S43.

17. Bartocci M, Winberg J, Ruggiero C, Bergqvist LL, Serra G, Lagercrantz H. Activation of olfactory cortex in newborn infants after odor stimulation: a functional near-infrared spectroscopy study. *Pediatr Res* 2000; 48: 18-23.

18. Bartocci M, Winberg J, Papendieck G, Mustica T, Serra G, Lagercrantz H. Cerebral hemodynamic response to unpleasant odors in the preterm newborn measured by near-infrared spectroscopy. *Pediatr Res* 2001; 50: 324-30.

19. Hintz SR, Benaron DA, Siegel AM, Zourabian A, Stevenson DK, Boas DA. Bedside functional imaging of the premature infant brain during passive motor activation. *J Perinat Med* 2001; 29: 335-43.

20. Bucher HU, Moser T, von Siebenthal K, Keel M, Wolf M, Duc G. Sucrose reduces pain reaction to heel lancing in preterm infants: a placebo-controlled, randomized and masked study. *Pediatr Res* 1995; 38: 332-5.

Is it necessary to prove that developmental care is beneficial?

Gorm Greisen

Should babies be treated with respect for their developmental needs and personal integrity? Should parents be allowed to stay with their baby and to participate in care and in decisions? These are questions of value. These questions can not be answered by experience, but must include other perspectives. The good of the developmental care concept is a moral question, but the costs and risks of applying these concepts are not.

Who has the burden of proof? Some institutions already have formal individualised developmental care as the backbone of their services; others have humanised various aspects of care; others look at it as a luxury, and still others regard it with suspicion as a threat to effective medical treatment. When must a practice have an explicit rationality?

Firstly, *those doing more than others should know why*. A basic principle in medicine is "first, do no harm". Anything which can have a beneficial effect is, by necessity, also capable of doing harm. I believe this is true of medical care using surgery or drugs. Even a simple thing, however, such as being more aware of the baby's signs of discomfort during turning him from side to side means, in principle, being less aware of the position of the tracheal tube.

Secondly, *the "unnatural" and the "new" has a case to answer*. Nature has a track record of optimising long term benefits in the form of the survival of our species. Being natural, however, is not a wholesale argument for being good. Nature has provided man with excess fertility, and part of the natural human program is a significant loss of young children. Medical traditions also have records, although the records are often poorly kept. Furthermore it is often unclear which parts of a medical practice that are essential and which parts are nonessential or even harmful. Dimming light and reducing noise is natural, but can possibly lead to less accurate observation of physical signs and less precise communication among the care team members.

Thirdly, *interventions that are invasive, potentially dangerous, painful, or just unpleasant must serve a well defined purpose*. Here traditional neonatal care has much to defend, but developmental care attempting developmentally adjusted stimulation may fall within this category.

Finally, *interventions which use extra human or economic resources must be defended*. The provision of health care falls further and further behind its potentials as medical science advances faster than the economical growth. This is true in affluent as well as less affluent societies. In the context of developmental care, the attention and time used by parents does not represent increased use of resources, it may even reduce anxiety and psychological stress. But the time used by staff is costly, and it is necessary to consider cost-effectiveness.

Reductionist approach

We have good assumptions about the inner working of the body and mind as well as about the steps in the natural course of events. Therefore, intermediate end-points are important. Looking for better ways of reducing pain and stress and improving cardiorespiratory stability, feeding and growth, and psychomotor development in the short term is useful before testing for definite benefits is carried out in large scale randomised controlled trials.

Randomised controlled trials

The methodology of the randomised and controlled trial (RCT) is the cornerstone of modern medical science. It is based on the assumption that diseases and processes of disease exist, not only in ill people. It assumes that the course of illness in two patients may be meaningfully compared and that if the choice of treatment is made at random, then any systematic difference in outcome between patients treated differently may soundly lead to the conclusion that the treatments differ as to their effects. If treatments are not chosen at random, differences in outcome may be ascribed to the reasons for choosing the treatment as well as to the treatment as such. Nonmedical care professionals are often sceptical about the use of RCT to test the efficacy of their often highly individualised treatment. The central problem is to define a "control" or "reference" treatment against which a comparison is meaningful.

A recent meta-analysis reviews 32 RCTs of various interventions labelled developmental care including a total of more than 2000 babies [1]. Another 46 studies were excluded. Interventions were grouped into categories such as positioning, modification of external stimuli, and individualized developmental care interventions. The most consistent benefits were found for individualized developmental care interventions with reduction of ventilatory support (- 1 week for mechanical ventilation, and - 5 weeks for supplementary oxygen), shorter hospital stay (- 2 weeks), and better psychomotor development (+ 1 standard deviation score). These are very important benefits. However, some important methodological problems limit the strength of the conclusions and precludes recommendations for clinical practice.

It is important to examine studies from a methodological perspective. First, the end-point, or the primary effect of an RCT must be simple and chosen *a-priori*. All of the reviewed studies reported multiple outcomes. No more than three studies could be included in the estimation of the magnitude of the benefit regarding any outcome. Secondly, half of the RCTs had methodological problems related to blinding. Blinding is important to reduce the risk that preconceptions about the effect of treatment will bias the evaluation of results. Results which require an element of subjective judgement, as frequently used in developmental research, is particularly prone to bias. Thirdly, each RCT enrolled only a small number of babies. RCTs with small numbers of patients, on the average, yields larger treatment effects than RCTs with large number of patients. A major reason for this is likely to be "publication bias", that is, it is more likely that a RCT will be published if the result is positive. It is therefore a problem that the few RCTs of developmental care involved relatively small numbers of babies and showed statistically significant, *i.e.* large beneficial effects, even when one could expect the effects to be small-to-intermediate.

New randomised controlled trials

Equipoise, or a balance of pro's and con's, must exist for randomisation to be justifiable. Equipoise is partly subjective, since the relative weight of the pros and cons is personal, therefore parents as well as caretakers must be asked. Randomised controlled trials of developmental care as a concept is unfeasible, because it is not possible to explain to parents nor to staff, why some babies should be cared for without protection against pain and stress, without respect for their individual needs, or by less experienced staff.

Different methods of developmental care, on the other hand, may have sufficient equipoise to be compared by randomised controlled trials. The conclusion from meta-analysis stresses that a single primary end-point of clinical relevance must be chosen. The best candidate is psychomotor outcome at 2 years of age. Trials must be designed with sufficient power and with sufficient guards against bias, to insure that the enthusiasm of the investigators, wanting to prove the value of what they believe is the best, to spill over on outcome is avoided. Testing should involve a variety of social, cultural, and neonatal care settings. Costs must be assessed directly during implementation and maintenance.

Hermeneutic approach

Human activity is the subject for hermeneutic research. Hermeneutic methods may be used to relate the various aspects of neonatal care to the societal value of the very preterm baby and to parental roles in general and the mother-child relation in particular.

A basic assumption is that the researcher has an innate, human ability to understand his object of study, that he can differentiate the meaningful from the meaningless. Hermeneutic research leads to descriptions of which one part is the object under research and the other part is the researcher himself, by means of his pre-existing conceptualisations. The description and its interpretation are interlinked. The quality, or trueness, of the interpretation depends on its completeness, its explanatory power, and its ability to resolve apparent contradictions. In hermeneutic research there is no account of random variation. Many aspects of developmental care research are well suited to hermeneutic methods. The behaviour of babies, parents and staff can be described and interpreted with scientific rigour, and it would be unreasonable to replace good qualitative research by bad randomised controlled trials.

Conclusion

The concept of developmental care requires moral reflection on practice, not documentation. Methods of developmental care require documentation of non-inferiority only, when it is less invasive, more natural, simpler and cheaper than conventional care. When it is formal, demanding, or interferes with effective provision of conventional care and treatment it requires evidence of superiority.

References

1. Symington A, Pinelli J. *Developmental care for promoting development and preventing morbidity in preterm infants* (Cochrane Review). In: The Cochrane Library, Issue 1. Chichester, UK: John Wiley & Sons Ltd, 2004.

Points of interest for future research

Björn Westrup, Hugo Lagercrantz

Developmental care of the prematurely born infant is a unique caregiving routine unique since it takes place during a critical period of life when the development of the brain is extremely active. Even if most of the neuronal migration has already taken place, there is a very active synthesis, migration, organisation and transformation of oligodendroglia, astrocytes and other white matter cells. Programmed neuronal cell death (apoptosis), dendritic formation and synaptogenesis are all essential activities in brain development that happens during this period. These activities are not only determined by genes but to a substantial degree are influenced by sensory input to the infant [1]. The environment and caregiving practices may have a major impact on brain development of the prematurely born infant by triggering transcription factors and thus potentially affect long-term development.

Moreover, long-term outcomes have been shown to be influenced by a well-functioning parent-child relationship [2-5]. A prematurely born infant behaves differently in comparison with a term infant. Consequently, the caregiving is more demanding and requires special skills. It would be of interest to investigate whether developmental care would support parents and other caregivers in their ability to meet these needs.

Finally, from an ethical point of view, family centred developmentally supportive care is of great interest. As far as we know there is no other well defined programme which in an equally thorough way teaches parents and caregivers the language of the prematurely born infant. Just as patients with a different native tongue than the prevailing language of the country providing the care these patients are entitled to interpreters, *i.e.*, developmentally trained personnel who readily can understand their subtle, non-verbal way of communication. Guidance and training in this could also be considered a right of the parents [6-9].

Research on individualised developmentally supportive care

Evaluating the effects of individualised developmental intervention programs, such as NIDCAP (Newborn Individualised Developmental Care and Assessment Program) is complicated. In comparison to drug trials it is extremely difficult to achieve a standard experimental design in this kind of study. There is no gold standard for nursing care, making the definition of the control group variable. The intervention cannot be applied in a blinded fashion. The experiments may include several individual approaches, which provide confounding factors and a single procedure may not be analysed separately. The duration of integrated care procedures using the NIDCAP model lasts for the duration of the infant's hospital stay, often over several months, leading to a risk of spill over effect on the control group. Parents share experiences with each other and actively seek knowledge designed to improve the treatment of their infant.

The introduction of developmentally supportive care is a multidisciplinary process involving not only neuroscience and nursing, but also developmental psychobiology, family interventions and psychological approaches. NIDCAP implies physical changes in the NICU, as well as considerable educational efforts. To our knowledge, NIDCAP is the only program that encompasses a holistic view of the caregiving of the newborn infant, and which includes both an assessment of the infant and a presentation of individualised caregiving plan. Do we know the most appropriate approach for assessing such very early and complex intervention?

Thus, the researcher of developmental care will encounter a lack of understanding on different levels. First, the research institutions must realise that the design of developmental research project requires very careful planning with many disciplines involved. Second, there has to be quite an extensive pre-trial period of necessary training of staff planned to be involved in the implementation of the intervention. A related matter is retention of the highly trained nursing staff and assurance that they are "allowed" the assignments of observations as necessary throughout the study despite the staffing and the familiar economical problems.

Alas, should we give in to these problems and just let the development take its own course driven by individual, dedicated nurses and encouraged by the increasing and strong demand from parents of prematurely born infants?

We believe not. As scientists we have the obligation to assess this quite expensive programme to the best of our capacity. In addition, the question of possible adverse effects is not completely resolved at this time. The studies published so far have been few and with small numbers, *i.e.*, the power has been low and there is an obvious risk of type II errors, which could conceal negative as well as positive effects.

Published studies

There are two recent systematic reviews and meta-analyses on developmental care [10-11]. Both reviews indicate that individualised developmental care interventions (mainly NIDCAP) demonstrate improved growth outcomes, decreased respiratory support, decreased length and cost of hospital stay as well as improved neurodevelopmental outcomes up to 12 or 24 months. In addition Jacobs and collaborators found an indication of improved behaviour at term age. To our knowledge, there is no other intervention in the neonatal period reporting similar positive effects on such a number of important outcome variables. However, in both reviews there is a concern regarding the sizes of published studies as well as of some methodological shortcomings. They conclude that more high quality randomised controlled trials are warranted before a clear direction for practice can be supported. These trials should include consistent outcome variables assessed at consistent times in order to ameliorate problems for further meta-analyses. Assessment of the cost-benefit of the intervention is essential as well.

There are a number of other studies supporting the conclusions of the meta-analyses [12-15]. In addition, we have reported on improved behaviour and mother infant interaction at three years of age in a group of infants subjected to NIDCAP [16] and less distractibility and attention problems at a five-year follow-up [17].

Suggested areas for future investigations

Developmental studies of well-defined events

During the early postnatal period of an infant born very prematurely, there are many well-defined events that are commonly occurring and often experienced as challenging to the autonomic stability. Thus, it would be of great interest to study developmental interventions during, for example, diaper change, weighing, medical rounds, x-rays and eye examinations. Moreover, it would be of interest to further explore the impact of kangaroo-care in the early postnatal period.

Individualised developmental intervention programs

Large, possibly multi-centre, randomised trials are warranted in order to confirm the rather astonishing results of the published smaller trials. There should be a focus on long-term cognitive and behavioural outcome, *i.e.*, the assessments should continue until the children reach two, five or ten years of age. Secondary outcomes of interest could be short-term effects on growth, nutrition, lung morbidity, brain maturation and morbidity, infant behaviour and parent-infant interaction. Examples of methods that could be of interest to employ are displayed in *table 1*. Moreover, analyses of the cost-effectiveness are needed.

Although it is important to study possible effects in units with differences in medico-cultural contexts, it also implies a methodological challenge. In addition, the fairly small number of infants born very prematurely in each unit also makes a randomisation process hazardous. One way around these problems would be to randomise by site instead of by patient. However, such a procedure would demand at least four times as many subjects in order to achieve adequate power. In the light of the current shortage of developmentally skilled interveners, this is not feasible within the foreseeable future. Employing a semi- randomisation/stratification procedure such as minimisation [18] might be an acceptable compromise in this situation.

Another issue of concern is how to ascertain a contrast between the intervention and control group in units that have already implemented some sort of individualised care for many years. Could the control group in these units really be considered as conventionally treated? On the other hand, it is definitely of interest to assess if the full implementation of a complex program as NIDCAP is needed in order to get an impact on the well being of the infants. Again, some sort of regionalization might be useful in a multi-centre trial.

Table I. Assessment tools of interest.

Autonomic regulation	Respiratory control (apnoeas) MAP (mean arterial blood pressure)
Stress response	Salivary cortisol HRV (Heart Rate Variability)
Brain maturation and function	MRI (Magnetic Resonance Imaging) DTI (Diffusion Tensor Imaging) NIRS (Near Infra Red Spectroscopy) BEAM (Brain Electrical Area Mapping) Cortical coherence
Parent health	PSI (Parental Stress Index) EPDS (Edinburgh Postnatal Depression Scale)
Cognition and behaviour	BSID-II (Bayley Scale of Infant Development-II) WPPSI-R (Wechsler Preschool and Primary Scale of Intelligence – Revised)

The implementation process

The surveillance of the implementation process of developmental care is crucial in order to ascertain the quality of the intervention. What is the level of awareness and training among the staff in general and among the caregivers for the intervention of infants in particular? How is the physical environment in the NICU for respective groups? How intense was the intervention? How many behavioural observations were performed per each infant? In addition, could the number of behavioural observations per full time employee in the unit indicate the degree of implementing developmental care in the unit?

Furthermore, the costs of the intervention must be recorded, *e.g.*, staff time, training fees, staff time for observations, as well as cost of the actual care for each infant such as days in intensive care or hospital charges.

Next step

Developmental care provides great potential in playing an important role in modern neonatology. With increased collaboration among researchers in the field of developmental care, we believe it is important that we proceed with determining if individualised developmental care is warranted in modern NICUs. There is a need for collaborative studies and joint efforts in getting adequate funding. The training process and guidance in implementation of individualised developmental care requires co-ordination and an organisational platform. Moreover, there is a need of disseminating the findings of present research and future directions in this field to the rest of the communities of neonatology and follow-up.

References

1. *The newborn brain.* Lagercrantz H, Hanson M, Evrard P, Rodeck C, eds. Cambridge: Cambridge University Press, 2002, 538 p.

2. Devitto B, Goldberg S. The effects of newborn medical status on early parent-infant interaction. In: Field TM, Soslek AM, Goldberg S, Shuman HH, eds. *Infants Born at Risk. Behavior and Development.* New York: Spectrum, 1979: 311-32.

3. Bakeman R, Brown JV. Early interaction: consequences for social and mental development at three years. *Child Dev* 1980; 51: 437-47.

4. Field TM. Interactions of high-risk infants: quantative and qualitative differences. In: Sawin DB, Hawkins EC, Walker LO, Penticuff JM, eds. *Psychosocial Risks in Infants.* New York: Brunner/Mazel, 1980: 120-43.

5. Minde K, Whitelaw A, Brown J, Fitzhardinge P. Effect of neonatal complications in premature infants on early parent-infant interactions. *Dev Med Child Neurol* 1983; 25: 763-77.

6. Levin A. Humane Neonatal Care Initiative. *Acta Paediatr* 1999; 88: 353-5.

7. Kennell JH. The Humane Neonatal Care Initiative. *Acta Paediatr* 1999; 88: 367-70.

8. Sizun J, Ratynski N, Boussard C. Humane Neonatal Care Initiative, the NIDCAP and the Family-Centered Neonatal Intensive Care. *Acta Paediatr* 1999; 88: 1172.

9. Westrup B, Kleberg A, Stjernqvist K. The Humane Neonatal Care Initiative and family-centred developmentally supportive care. *Acta Paediatr* 1999; 88: 1051-2.

10. Jacobs SE, Sokol J, Ohlsson A. The Newborn Individualized Developmental Care and Assessment Program is not supported by meta-analyses of the data. *J Pediatr* 2002; 140: 699-706.

11. Pinelli J, Symington A. Non-nutritive sucking for the promotion of physiologic stability and nutrition in preterm infant. *Cochrane Database Syst Rev* 2001; 3: CD 001071.

12. Parker SJ, Zahr LK, Cole JG, Brecht ML. Outcome after developmental intervention in the neonatal intensive care unit for mothers of preterm infants with low socioeconomic status. *J Pediatr* 1992; 120: 780-5.

13. Becker PT, Grunwald PC, Moorman J, Stuhr S. Effects of developmental care on behavioral organization in very-low-birth-weight infants. *Nurs Res* 1993; 42: 214-20.

14. Stevens B, Petryshen P, Hawkins J, Smith B, Taylor P. Developmental *versus* conventional care: A comparison of clinical outcomes for very low birth weight infants. *Can J Nurs Res* 1996; 28: 97-113.

15. Brown LD, Heermann JA. The effect of developmental care on preterm infant outcome. *Appl Nurs Res* 1997; 10: 190-7.

16. Kleberg K, Westrup B, Stjernqvist K. Developmental outcome, child behaviour and mother and child interaction, at three years following NIDCAP® (Newborn Individualized Developmental Care and Assessment Program) intervention. *Early Hum Dev* 2000; 60: 123-35.

17. Westrup B, Böhm B, Lagercrantz H, Stjernqvist K. Preschool outcome in children born very preterm and cared according to NIDCAP. *Acta Paediatr* 2004; 93: 498-507.

18. Altman DG. *Practical statistics for medical research.* London: Chapman & Hall; 1991.

Achevé d'imprimer par Corlet, Imprimeur, S.A.
14110 Condé-sur-Noireau
N° d'Imprimeur : 87729 - Dépôt légal : décembre 2005

Imprimé en France